T0264960

Income Generation in General Practice

ANDREW A.F. SANDERSON

General Practitioner, Spennymoor,
County Durham

RADCLIFFE MEDICAL PRESS
OXFORD

© 1991 Radcliffe Medical Press Ltd.
15 Kings Meadow, Ferry Hinksey Road, Oxford OX2 0DP

All rights reserved. No part of this publication may be reproduced,
stored in a retrieval system, or transmitted, in any form or by any means,
electronic, mechanical, photocopying, recording or otherwise
without the prior permission of the copyright owner.

British Library Cataloguing in Publication Data

Sanderson, Andrew F.
  Income generation in general practice.
  1. General practice. Finance
  I. Title
362.170905
ISBN 1-870905-02-4

Typeset by Advance Typesetting Ltd, Oxford
Printed and bound in Great Britain by TJ Press Ltd, Padstow, Cornwall

Contents

	Acknowledgements	v
	Preface	vii
1	Basic Practice Allowance	1
2	Temporary Residents	5
3	Night Visits and Out of Hours Services	7
4	Contraception	9
5	Maternity Medical Services	11
6	Screening	19
7	Child Health Surveillance	21
8	Health Promotion Clinics	23
9	Target Payments	25
10	Vaccinations and Immunizations	31
11	Minor Surgery	33
12	Rural Practice Payments	35
13	Dispensing	37
14	Postgraduate Education Allowance	41
15	Training	43
16	Premises	49
17	Improvement Grants	59
18	Employing Staff	61
19	Computer Costs	65
20	Sickness & Maternity Payments	67
21	The Practice Accountant	69
22	Non-National Health Service Work	81
23	Petty Cash	87
24	Expenditure	89
25	Joining a Practice	95
	Index	99

Acknowledgements

THERE are a number of people who I would like to thank for their help towards this book. Firstly my family who have put up with my typing and printer late into the night. Secondly my partner Alan Sensier, my friend David Elleanor and my accountant Peter Willey who all did proof-reading and offered valuable advice. Next to thank are my trainees, for whom the project was originally started. Finally Kenneth Clarke, former Secretary of State, who irritated me sufficiently to finish the book.

ANDREW F. SANDERSON

Preface

GENERAL practice as we have been told many times is a business, and businesses are there to generate income. There is plenty of advice on the clinical aspect of general practice, and some on management in the speciality, but the only advice on generating income is to be found in the free journals and newspapers. The object of this book is to put together general advice for those new to general practice so that they do not spend years working hard and not taking the rewards owing to them.

I do not pretend to provide comprehensive instructions on every possible route to income generation – that would take a multi-volume textbook. This book can only contain general advice with some specific clarification of the Statement of Fees and Allowances (the Red Book), as it is the Red Book which controls our income.

Throughout the book I have used the masculine to refer to a general practitioner (GP). This is purely for brevity, and is not meant to slight female GPs. Indeed, having two sisters who have been in practice, I dare not.

It has been said that the good GP will each night read a chapter of the Bible and a chapter of the Red Book. Certainly each GP should, if he wants full reward for his labours, have an up-to-date copy of the Red Book. Failure to read and understand this document before starting a new project has cost most GPs some income and has cost some of us a great deal of money. Witness the practitioner who decided to build new premises, without Red Book advice. He apparently appointed an architect who designed a surgery whose cost was many tens of thousands of pounds more than was allowed under the regulations. After finding out the awful truth, the architect was instructed to bring the cost within the tight limits permitted, but he was unable to do so. The episode finished with the doctor having lots of plans but no building. He also still had to pay the architect approaching £20,000 in fees for which there was no reimbursement.

General considerations

Several times each year, the medical press contains reports of the deliberations of the General Medical Council. Several of these are stories of doctors who have tried to defraud their patients, other doctors, the Family Health Services Authority (FHSA) or the Inland Revenue. Excepting moral considerations, fraud is stupid. A doctor earns by legitimate means from medical practice say £30,000 per year, and will continue to do so for the rest of his working life, if he behaves. If he then tries to get a few hundred or thousand more by underhand methods he is liable to lose his job and with it his earning potential and also much of his pension. Getting a new job in general practice after being found guilty of fraud will be difficult, what do you put on your CV? It would be extremely foolish to tempt fate in this manner.

There are ethical points which ought to be made. Patients put their trust in GPs and we cannot afford to abuse that trust.

Similarly the government, as the employing contractor, is owed value for money. In consequence we ought to spend taxpayers' money with care. We may make more income by using a higher priced treatment; but it is immoral to give an expensive treatment when a cheaper one will do equally well.

Talking to some doctors, it may seem that their income is above average, despite the fact that they drive a 5-year-old Ford Escort and live in a hovel. It may be that when speaking of their income, they have forgotten about the expenses portion of the money which comes from the FHSA.

When our remuneration is calculated by the Review Body, there are two parts to their deliberations. They have to decide upon the average pay for a GP, and then work out the approximate cost to him of running his practice for the current year. The latter is classed as expenses, is not superannuable, and is added to the former. This is why, when you look at the slips from the FHSA, the gross amount payable and the superannuable income are different.

'To tax and to please, no more than to love and to be wise, is not given to men' (Edmund Burke). Nevertheless we have to pay taxes. The trick is to make them as painless as possible. I have met a GP who pretends that taxes do not exist and twice a year is presented with a nasty reminder which takes 2 months' pay to cover. Your accountant should be able to estimate your tax liability for the current year, so that you can put aside sufficient money each month to cover the tax bill. It may be more appropriate to do this as a practice rather than as individuals, remembering that in a partnership you are liable for your partners' debts. Thus if your partner does not pay his tax, the man from the Inland Revenue will come to you for his money.

Much of the income coming from an FHSA to a partnership may be dependent upon there being a partnership as defined by the regulations. To have a partnership, the largest share of income from the practice must not be more than three times the smallest. This may seem to be easy, but on occasions it can be a problem. Take a partnership of three where two partners have parity of 36% and a new partner joined a year ago on 28% for 2 years. This practice then takes on a part-time partner doing no night shifts, but 25 hours a week to ensure a basic practice allowance. The agreement is that the new partner should have 10%. The existing partners would take 32%, 32% and 28%. They no longer have a partnership in the eyes of the FHSA. Some other arrangement must be made so that the two on parity are not getting more than three times the share of the part-timer. A solution could be to give the junior partner in the old practice parity.

As well as this, each partner must do a reasonable share of general medical services. You cannot have one partner who spends most of his time doing private or sessional work outside the practice, or who is semi-retired. This can be a trap for the woman in practice with her husband.

In some areas a FHSA may require a certificate from an independent solicitor stating that a partnership agreement conforming to certain criteria exists.

ANDREW SANDERSON
March 1991

1 Basic Practice Allowance
(SFA paragraphs 12.1–20.4)

THE basic practice allowance (BPA). (SFA para. 12.1–18.12) currently provides the average GP with about 20% of his income. It is important that the conditions set down in the Red Book are fulfilled, as the local FHSA has the power to withdraw some or all of the basic practice allowance payable to a doctor if they are not. Essentially, the conditions require the doctor to have 1200 patients on his list, and to devote a substantial part of his time to his practice. The latter part is defined as an average over the year of 26 hours per week. The time spent in the practice must also be spread over 5 days, so you cannot cram your 26 hours into 1 or 2 days. There are provisions in the Red Book and your terms of service for those who want to work less time. You can work more than 26 hours spread over 4 days if you are doing some other 'health related activity' on th 5th day. If you do not want to work 26 hours, you can work between 19 and 26 hours (three-quarters time). You can work between 13 and 19 hours (half-time). Alternatively you can share a full-time job with someone else. The amount of BPA money you get, will depend upon the time you spend in the practice.

Within a practice, each partner does not have to have 1200 patients, as long as the partnership has an average of 1200 per doctor. Here you must ensure that you have a partnership as is defined in the regulations.

There are some additions to the BPA which are available. The amount of money you get is proportional to the amount of basic practice allowance received.

The designated area allowance (SFA para. 14.1–14.11) is paid to doctors working in an underdoctored area. There are two levels of designation. Level 1 is paid when an area has had at least 3000 patients per doctor for at least 3 years. Level 2 is paid when the area has had 3000 patients per doctor for at least 1 year. You can graduate from level 2 to level 1.

Seniority payments (SFA para. 16.1–17) are, along with the postgraduate education allowance, the payments most commonly retained by individual doctors rather than paid into the practice. These are gained by being registered for the appropriate length of time. You also need to be a GP with full basic practice allowance for a lesser period (11 years registered and 7 years GP for first seniority, 18 years registered and 14 years GP for second seniority, 25 years registered and 21 years GP for third seniority). The date of registration is taken as the date of provisional registration. If you work as an assistant, each 2 years will count as 1 year towards seniority.

There is now an addition to the basic practice allowance to help you employ an assistant. To qualify you need 3000 patients for the first doctor in your practice, and 2500 for each subsequent doctor. A half-time assistant can be employed for half the money, requiring 2500 patients per partner. If you qualify for a rural practice payment, you may need fewer patients.

Associate allowance

This allows two or more single-handed practitioners to employ a doctor to allow the principals to have holiday time and time for postgraduate training. To get the allowance, you must be getting a rural practice payment, or be sole doctors on an island. You must also be getting an inducement payment, or have at least 10 miles from your surgery to the local hospital. *Remember* that an associate is an employee, and pays tax under the PAYE arrangements.

How much you pay an associate is up to you, but the amount you get from the FHSA is fixed. You will be allowed annual increments, National Insurance contributions, a car allowance and an allowance for a telephone. The associate may be able to get expenses for removal, storage of furniture, house purchase and house sale. An associate can also qualify for the postgraduate training allowance.

If you do get an associate allowance, you cannot get locum fees reimbursed. If you and your associate part company, and he is paid in lieu of notice, you can get up to 1 month's worth of that pay reimbursed.

Deprivation allowance

GPs providing services to deprived areas (as measured by the Jarmen index) are paid a supplement to the BPA in respect of all patients on their lists who live in areas categorized as 'deprived'. Each patient living in a deprived area will attract a BPA supplement.

GPs with individual or average partnership lists of less than 400 patients, and therefore not in receipt of BPA, still qualify for deprivation payments for all patients on their lists living in deprived areas.

There are three payment bands, and it is the Secretary of State who decides on deprived area definitions. He gets his information from the most recent national census. The next one is due in the next 18 months. After this, areas of deprivation may change.

Leave payment

This is an interest-free loan or advance on the BPA. You must apply by 15 April but it is best to apply early, perhaps in January. Organize a holiday of at least a week in April or early May and this is the one upon which you claim. The FHSA will send you a cheque for one fifth of your BPA, probably on 1 April. The money will be deducted from your quarterly payments (June, September, December and March) over the next year. You can use it to finance anything you like, a holiday, a new dining room table, or even put it in the bank (high-interest deposit account), gaining interest until you need it.

2 Temporary Residents
(SFA paragraphs 32.1 – 9) (FP19, FP1003)

A temporary resident is defined as a patient who is in your area for at least 24 hours, but not more than 3 months. There are two rates payable, the lower for a patient resident for up to 15 days from the date on which the GP first provides treatment, and the higher for the temporary resident expecting to stay for more than 15 days.

Where the only treatment provided attracts an item of service fee for vaccination, immunization, contraceptive services, maternity medical services or the arrest of dental haemorrhage, only the fee for that item is payable and not the temporary resident fee. It should be remembered that fees are only payable if the patient is temporarily resident in the area; fees cannot be claimed for patients who are permanently resident in the area but whom a GP wishes to accept only on a temporary basis.

Where you are in an area which attracts a lot of visitors, you can get advances on your temporary resident fees, a move which will improve your cash flow.

Contraception for visitors is claimed separately with FP1003 (which will be one-quarter of the annual fee), and if you give a woman temporary resident contraceptive advice and general medical services, you can claim both FP19 and FP1003.

Emergency treatment
(SFA 33.1 – 10) (FP32)

Where the visitor is in your area for less than 24 hours you must treat him if treatment is necessary. The claim however is made for emergency treatment. This is worth more than a temporary resident.

If you have to treat a person living in your area who is on the list of another practice then you claim under emergency treatment, and the FHSA will ask the other doctor why he was not available, and if his answer if not reasonable, the fee will be deducted from him.

If the cause of the emergency is a road – traffic accident, you must if possible invoice the injured person's insurance company, because payment will not be made by the FHSA unless this action has tried and failed.

Immediately necessary treatment (SFA 36.1 – 7)   (FP106)

This is for people who need urgent treatment and who live in your practice area either permanently or as temporary residents. However, you do not wish to have them on your list. It also covers the situation where you are appealing against a patient's assignment to your list. Where it is appropriate, you can also claim a maternity fee, a fee for arrest of dental haemorrhage and a night visit fee.

If they subsequently join your or your partner's list, payment is made from the date that you gave the original urgent treatment.

3 Night Visit Fees and Out of Service Hours Services
(SFA paragraph 24.1–7)

'OUT of hours' is defined as 8.00pm to 8.00am. You get an item of service fee for each visit **requested and made** to a patient on your list or as a temporary resident between 10.00pm and 8.00am. Generally the visit will be at the patient's home, but there are exceptions. So if a call comes in at 7.45am but you do not stir yourself until 8.15am, you do not get the fee. Similarly, a call at 9.55pm, does not qualify for the fee. Do not be tempted to claim, as the FHSA has the right to check (with the patient) on your night claims, and will do so at random.

If you see two patients (not a mother and new baby) on one visit to one address you get twice the money. More than that at one visit will also give you more money. Patients three to five will give you an extra half fee each. More than that will only give you one tenth of a fee each! If you think that you have been cheated, write to the FHSA and they may give you more.

There are two levels of payment. You get the higher level if the visit is made by the patient's registered doctor or that doctor's partner or another doctor from the same group practice. The call can be made by an assistant, deputy, locum or trainee of the group. This assumes that the trainee has done at least 3 months in general practice. If you employ a deputy directly, inform the FHSA of his employment, and if he does the visit, the higher fee is payable. If however it is the deputizing service (or a trainee who has not done the 3 months) then only the lower fee is payable. You can also get the higher fee if you are in a non-commercial rota of 10 or less. Remember to let the FHSA know the names of those on the rota.

4 Contraception
(SFA paragraphs 29.1–12) (FP1001, FP1002, FP1003)

CONTRACEPTION is a steady source of income for most GPs. It is not difficult to follow the rules.

The fee is payable for contraceptive **advice**, and any necessary examination. The prescription of the pill, cap, etc., is not essential, although if your advice is to take the pill and the woman agrees, then the prescription is part of the service. You can also claim if you help the patient choose a method of contraception and accept responsibility for any necessary aftercare. This means that if a woman attends the surgery and advice is given about a male contraceptive or vasectomy, a GP can still claim if they accept responsibility for the aftercare of the female patient.

The fee is payable in four equal amounts at the end of each quarter. If you fit an intrauterine device, a fitting fee is also payable and is paid in the first quarter, so at the end of the first quarter after fitting a coil you will get the fitting fee and one quarter of the ordinary annual contraceptive fee.

It is essential that you keep good records of not only your advice and treatment, but of the date that you last obtained the woman's signature on an FP1001. This is for two reasons, firstly, 11 months must have elapsed since a previous form was signed before a new signature is valid. If you do get a new FP1001 signed, it will be valid from the date that the previous one expired. Secondly, if you are late with the form (up to 18 months from the first claim), by correctly completing part 4 on the back of the form, arrears can be paid by the FHSA. These arrears are for quarters for which you have given contraceptive services since the previous FP1001 expired. Remember to send in your correctly filled in and signed forms to the FHSA on a regular basis.

Example

1990	1991
J F M A M J J A S O N D	J F M A M J J A S O N D
1	2 3 4

1 – Claim made on FP1001
2 – Earliest next claim on FP1001
3 – Date when next FP1001 is due, and from which early claims are valid
4 – Last date to be able to get continuous payment with back credits.

Early in each quarter you will be notified of the number of women for whom there are current claims, and also the number for whom you have fitted a coil in the previous quarter. You will see the arrears appear on your FHSA contraceptive list size sheets as back credits. You should keep a record of the number of current FP1001s and FP1002s so that if the FHSA records are incorrect you can challenge them. If you want to challenge the FHSA returns, you have only 10 days in which to do so. This is your only opportunity.

5   Maternity Medical Services
(SFA paragraphs 31.1–19 and schedule 1,2,3)(FP24)

MATERNITY is well-paid, well-understood and easy to claim properly, but it is also easy to lose out on payments if you are not vigilant.

The number of GPs providing full maternity services for their patients seems to be becoming less, but with increasing pressure from women wanting home-delivery and the large number of vocationally trained doctors who have done an obstetric job, this trend may be reversed.

The responsibilities for maternity medical services (MMS) are listed in the Red Book paragraph 31, schedule 1. The expected standards of care are in paragraph 31, schedule 3.

A doctor *not* on the Obstetric List who is providing these services will be paid a much lower level of fees than a doctor who is included. The obstetrically approved doctor can accept women for maternity services who are not on his ordinary list. To qualify for the Obstetric List you must have experience in obstetrics approved by the Local Obstetric Committee or the Secretary of State for Health.

Ante-natal care

There are three levels of fee payable. These are not affected if the patient receives any hospital care. They are paid if she is confined after the 28th week, or earlier if a live birth results. The levels are:

- a woman booking up the 16th week of pregnancy
- a woman booking from the 17th to 30th week of pregnancy
- a woman booking from the 31st week of pregnancy.

The date of booking is taken as the date the woman signs Part II of form FP24/24A. It is important for this and other reasons to ask your patient to sign the FP24 at the earliest opportunity.

Miscarriage

A miscarriage fee is paid for any maternity services provided if a woman's pregnancy ends during or before 28th week and does not result in a live birth.

Termination of pregnancy

If the patient has a termination after being accepted for maternity services, a miscarriage fee is paid for maternity services given prior to this decision. Post-operative care after an abortion does *not* qualify for post-natal care fees.

Confinement

This is paid for providing maternity services during a confinement, and includes GPs who provide care during labour for a patient who is not booked for maternity services with the GP.

Post-natal care

A *complete* post-natal care fee is paid if you provide maternity services to a mother and child for the 14 days immediately after confinement and carry out a full post-natal examination at or about 6 weeks after confinement. The complete fee will still be paid to you if the woman is confined in a hospital other than a GP unit, provided the woman leaves it not later than the second day after delivery.

A *partial* fee is paid if you provide care to mother and child during the 14 days after the birth. A separate fee is available for a full post-natal examination done between 6 and 12 weeks after confinement. The fee payable for five post-natal consultations and a full post-natal examination is the same as that available for complete post-natal care.

Remember that if the patient is confined at home or in a hospital and requires medical attendance beyond the 14th day you should provide this as part of your general medical services.

A useful fact to know is that if you are unable to carry out the post-natal examination but otherwise have provided complete care, the FHSA may pay the full fee if it is satisfied that you have made 'reasonable efforts' to carry out the examination. A 'reasonable effort' could include two letters from the GP to the patient requesting attendance at the surgery followed by either a request to the patient through the midwife, or a call by the doctor at the patient's home.

Complete maternity services fee

The complete maternity services fee is paid if you provide complete maternity services during pregnancy, confinement, the post-natal period and carry out a full post-natal examination at or about 6 weeks after confinement. You are entitled to the appropriate fees even if you refer the patient for a second opinion.

Anaesthetic

An anaesthetic fee is paid if, whilst you are providing maternity services, you call a second GP to give an anaesthetic.

Maternity services from another doctor

If a patient of yours receives care from another GP either temporarily or permanently after registering for maternity services with you then your fee will be limited to either the complete fee or a smaller amount appropriate to the actual services provided. See Figure 1 for clarification of this.

Figure 1: Example of apportionment of fees between two GPs providing maternity services to one woman

Both GPs on the Obstetric List

Expected date of confinement 16 October 1990

Dr A: Patient booked for MMS 25 April 1990 (15th week)
       Patient subsequently moved temporarily
Dr B: Patient booked for MMS 5 July 1990 (25th week)
       Patient returned home 38th week
Dr A: Care during confinement on 15 October 1990
       + post-natal care
       + post-natal examination at 6th week after
       confinement

continued

Figure 1: *continued*

Payment for ante-natal care

		Dr A	Dr B
1st level Dr A: (15th week)		£19.60	
2nd level Dr A: 8/13 × £19.55		£12.03	
Dr B: 5/13 × £19.55 (25th week)			£ 7.52
3rd level Dr A: 2/9 × £39.15		£ 8.70	
Dr B: 7/9 × £39.15			£30.45
		£40.33	£37.97

Total payment made: £78.30

Payment for confinement and post-natal care

Dr A:

Care during confinement		£33.35
Complete post-natal: (i) 5 visits @ £4.45 during 14 days puerperium		£22.25
(ii) post-natal pelvic examination at or about the 6th week		£11.10
		£66.70

Dr A is paid	£107.03
Dr B is paid	£ 37.97
Total fees paid	£145.00

NB: For apportionment purposes of ante-natal:

1st level (£78.30 – £58.70)	£19.60
2nd level (£58.70 – £39.15)	£19.55
3rd level	£39.15
	£78.30

Claims for payment

Claims for payment must be made to the FHSA in which your patient lives. If you are on the Obstetric List form FP24 is completed and if not form FP24A. Part II of the form must be completed and signed by the patient and Part III by you, but Part II contains a special certificate if you attend a woman in an emergency and you consider it undesirable to ask for her signature.

Completion of claim forms

It is in yours and your FHSA's best interest if you complete accurately and submit promptly form FP24A. Most FHSAs now process MMS forms by computer so accuracy is very important. See Figure 2, page 17 for clarification of those sections that are most often queried.

It is worthwhile organizing a system to ensure that you and your partners claim all their maternity services fees. This could involve systems run by other members of the practice, however, in my practice we have a system whereby when a positive pregnancy test is confirmed, the woman's name and address is put onto a small card. This then goes to the partner responsible for maternity who has access to everyone's book of FP24s. He follows the pregnancy using the card to identify the woman. When she is booked the card goes into a chronological file, appearing again when she delivers and also when she has her post-natal examination. At each significant event a note is made on the card. All letters about the pregnancy go to this partner so that he can claim miscarriage, etc. promptly. This system allows you to chase-up women who default from their post-natal examination and makes sure that all claims are made correctly.

Mary Marshmallow (Dr Pratt) 1 Joker Terrace, Mackemville		
L.M.P.	15.2.90	
E.D.D.	22.11.90	
Confined	28.11.90	
Postnatal due	9.1.91	done 17.1.91
Claim made	19.1.91 (book 16w Comp PN care)	
Paid	30.3.91 (£111.85)	

After the pregnancy and all the work is done, claim promptly and accurately as overclaiming is an offence taken very seriously by FHSAs.

NATIONAL HEALTH SERVICE   MATERNITY MEDICAL SERVICES

PART I

(to be detached and given to the patient)

To ....

I accept your application to receive maternity medical services from me.

Your expected date of confinement is   ....

Date ....   Doctor's signature ....

PART II

PATIENT'S APPLICATION FOR SERVICES

(Tick appropriate box)

Dr. ....

A   I wish to receive maternity medical services from you. I have not made arrangements for these services with another doctor.

☐

B   I wish to receive maternity medical services from you. I have cancelled arrangements

made with Dr. ....

of   ....

☐

C   I wish to receive maternity medical services from you whilst temporarily residing at:

....

....

☐

I have made arrangements for maternity medical services in my home area with

Dr. ....

....

D   I have received maternity medical services from you in an emergency.

☐

Patient's full name ....
(in block letters)

Home address   ....

....

Former name ....   N.H.S. No. ❶ ....
or Date of Birth

Date ....   Patient's signature ....

DOCTOR'S CERTIFICATE

(EMERGENCY ATTENDANCE FOR MISCARRIAGE)

I certify that in the circumstances I thought it desirable, in the patient's interest, not to
ask her for a signature.

Date ....   Doctor's signature ....

Form FP24

MATERNITY BENEFITS

There are cash benefits for mothers under the National Insurance Scheme which must be claimed within certain time limits. You are strongly advised to get Leaflet N.I. 17A and the necessary claim form from your local Maternity and Child Health Clinic, or from your local Department of Health and Social Security office not later than 14 weeks before your baby is expected.

PRESCRIPTION CHARGES AND WELFARE MILK AND VITAMINS

An expectant mother can apply on Part 1 of the Certificate of Pregnancy (Form FW8) for a prescription charge exemption certificate covering the period of her pregnancy and until her child is one year old. Details are given on Part 2 of Form FW8 and in leaflet MV11 (obtainable from Post Offices, local Department of Health and Social Security offices and local Maternity and Child Health Clinics) of how to claim free milk and vitamins.

PART III
DOCTOR'S CERTIFICATE AND CLAIM FOR PAYMENT
(References are to paragraphs in the Statement of Fees and Allowances)

(Tick appropriate box)

I certify that ....   *(patient's name)*

(expected date of confinement   ❷   )   had a miscarriage on   ❸   ☐
                                                  was confined on   ☐

at home ....   ☐
In the GP Unit at   ❹   Hospital   ☐
In   Hospital   ☐

I further certify that I provided the services indicated below and that I had regard to and was guided by authoritative medical opinion as set out in paragraphs 31.2 and paragraph 31/Schedule 3.

(i) Complete Maternity Medical Services   ❺   Paras 31.7 to 31.8   ☐

(ii) Ante-natal care

Note: the date of booking is the date on which Parts I and II are completed

(a) Patient booked up to 16th week of pregnancy   Para 31.9   ☐

(b) Patient booked from 17th week to 30th week
    of pregnancy   Para 31.9   ☐

(c) Patient booked from 31st week of pregnancy   Para 31.9   ☐

(iii) Miscarriage   Para 31.10   ☐

(iv) Care during the confinement   ❼   Para 31.11   ☐

(v) Complete Post-Natal Care (Date of Hospital Discharge ❻   ) Para 31.12 ☐

(vi) Partial Post-Natal Care   Para 31.13   ☐

(a) date of each attendance

(b) date of full post-natal examination   ❽

(vii) Other services as described in the attached note   ☐

(viii) Date of last service to patient
(to be completed where only ante-natal care or only complete post-natal care is given).

I claim payment for the above services   ☐

I also claim payment for the employment as anaesthetist of Dr.   ☐
                                          Paras 31.15 to 31.16

Date   Doctor's signature

Fees approved for payment £

Figure 2 Key:

[1] please enter correct NHS number;

[2] please enter this date other than when claiming for postnatal care only;

[3] it is important that these dates are *clearly* entered as appropriate;

[4] please enter these sections correctly because different fees are payable;

[5] this section must be completed when complete care is provided;

[6] this section should be completed *only* when a woman has been confined at home or in a GP unit;

[7] this section should be completed *only* when a woman is confined in hospital (other than a GP unit) for less than 48 hours;

[8] this section should be completed when partial care is given.

6 Screening

Patients not seen within 3 years

THIS is a relatively new concept to many GPs and initially it can be difficult to understand how income for the practice can be generated. It is important to limit the time you spend on doing things that you feel are not of value to you or your patient. You have a contractual requirement for those between 16 and 75 that you have not seen in the previous 3 years. It is important therefore to make sure that you have a reliable method to record consultations. You must also be able to find out who has and who has not had a recorded consultation in the previous 1095 days. You must then invite the patient to come for an examination. How you phrase the letter or telephone call is up to you. The invitation must be recorded. If they do not come to see you, you are required to invite them again in a year's time.

I feel that if you are going to spend money and time contacting patients, it would be a waste not to make something positive from it. The patient may gain by meeting you or your nurse and having the opportunity to air a problem. You may gain by including him in a clinic session, at a later date. Do not forget that these examinations can be done by 'suitably qualified' non-medically trained staff. This is likely to be your practice nurse.

When patients are seen under your contractual obligations there are a number of things you must do. You must weigh them and measure their height and test their urine and blood pressure. You then have to give advice on life-style – diet, exercise, smoking and drinking. You must ask about housing, employment and other social circumstances. You must inquire about illnesses, immunizations, allergies, medication and hereditary diseases. You must also ask about tests for breast and cervical cancer. Remember to write it all down.

The amount of time you spend on this is up to you. But why not make sure that their immunizations are up to date – tetanus and polio. Where are they going for their holiday? Do they need your help there? Is he in a job which leaves him open to hepatitis, or even anthrax? If the patient is female, does she need contraceptive advice? If she does, then give it, and claim on FP1001. Indeed, has she had her smear? If not make sure that you arrange one for her, so that she is helping you to reach your target for smears.

Patients aged 75 and over

You should give patients over 75 a consultation and a home visit. You should record anything that appears to be affecting the patient's general health, including:

- sensory functions
- mobility
- mental condition
- physical condition including continence
- social environment
- use of medicines.

Why not ensure that the patient is up to date with tetanus vaccinations and that they all know where to get a 'flu jab in the autumn? Indeed why not load the visits into the autumn months and give the 'flu jab there and then?

Newly registered patients

Patients who have just joined (or been assigned to) your list must be offered a consultation within 28 days. Remember that the invitation must be in writing (or if made orally, confirmed in writing) and be recorded in the notes. You do not have to provide this consultation for new patients under 5 years of age or patients transferring from a partner's list who have participated in this type of consultation in the last 12 months.

Practice protocol

One way to encourage patients to attend a registration consultation is to have the letters of invitiation, with a practice brochure, available at the surgery reception desk. Welcoming and well-informed reception staff can make all the difference here. Do not forget that newly registered patients can be included in various clinics if you think it necessary after their registration medical.

7 Child Health Surveillance
(SFA paragraphs 22.1–6) (FP/CHS)

IF you want to provide child health surveillance and be paid for such services, you must be on the FHSA Child Health Surveillance List.

You are required to follow the guidelines set out by your FHSA. These will probably be a minimum examination done at set intervals. The idea is for all children to get some developmental care. It is hoped that treatable abnormalities will thus be identified.

Are you eligible?

You will receive a fee for each child under 5 years of age for when services are provided in accordance with the programme agreed between the FHSA and the District Health Authority (DHA) for the area in which you practise.

Child health surveillance patient list

This list is separate from your normal NHS list. It would seem most appropriate to get the mother to sign the FP/CHS form when you first see her after the child is born. You should always keep a register of these children on your list. Remember that the doctor who has the child for surveillance may or may not be the same as his GP.

Payment

There is one level of fee and this is paid automatically according to the information provided by you on form FP/CHS. Payment is made whether or not any particular service has been provided during the preceding quarter. Payment will stop once the child reaches 5 years of age.

Apart from the child health surveillance fee, there are other moneys available. Do not forget that whilst you have the children coming to your surgery, you can immunize them thus adding to your target payments. There are also the child's parents. Have they had their tetanus? Remember that polio is specifically payable for parents of children being immunized. Why not do the mother's post-natal examination in the baby clinic? You could give her contraceptive advice at the same time.

8 Health Promotion Clinics
(SFA paragraphs 30.1–4) (FP/HPC)

THESE are potentially a source of unlimited income.

Eligible clinics

Each FHSA can decide on which clinics qualify for payment. However, there are guidelines that must be adhered to:

- health promotion and illness prevention includes initial surveillance for disease, disability and other health problems; general advice and counselling on good health
- a clinic may cover more than one area but if it does only one fee will be paid
- day-care facilities do not qualify for payment
- clinics held wholly or partially for activities which are separately remunerated (e.g. ante-natal) will *not* qualify for payment
- a clinic should normally last at least 1 hour; be advertised to patients and be provided with an open appointment system, a group session or separate appointments
- attendance should usually be at least 10 – check with your FHSA for details.

Rolling clinics are available in some areas. These are clinics where the clientele come at different times and you tot them up. There may be conditions attached to your clinics (such as a protocol and audit). Make sure that you keep full and accurate records of all your work at all times.

Health promotion clinics usually qualifying for payment include:

- well-person
- anti-smoking
- alcohol
- diet
- exercise
- stress management
- heart disease prevention
- diabetes.

Remember your FHSA will be able to advise on eligibility.

9 Target Payments
(SFA paragraphs 25.1 – 26.9 and 28.1 – 13)
(FP/TPB, FP/TCC)

PAYMENTS for the immunization of children and cervical cytology used to be made for each eligible time that you did it. This system has been replaced by one of payments if you reach set targets. Work done but failing to reach the target will not be paid for. When it comes to targets, the word to remember is **Accuracy**. You need to be accurate in your practice lists. This not only includes the numbers of people, but also their dates of birth. Do not assume the FHSA list is always correct, it can be wrong. The problem we all face is that we are dealing with small numbers of people, particularly for childhood immunizations. This problem has been eased since the Government agreed to calculate the targets on the practice list as a whole, rather than as separate lists for each partner.

Accuracy is also vital in the recording of procedures. If you do a smear or an immunization and it is not recorded properly, you may lose the payment for the procedure, or even worse, miss your target.

For both of these activities there are two target levels. Immunizing children is set at 70% and 90% of the number of courses needed to achieve full immunization of all eligible children on your list, cervical cytology 50% and 80%. You get the full fee for reaching the higher target, and a third of that fee for the lower target. It is very important to remember that the day that counts is the first day of each quarter.

Immunizing children

Children aged 2 and under

Children aged 2 and under are defined as children who were born from the 2nd day of the same quarter 3 years earlier and the 1st day of the corresponding quarter 1 year later. So your target population for the quarter January – March 1991 will include all the children born from 2 January 1988 to 1 January 1989 inclusive. The quarters begin on 1 January, 1 April, 1 July and 1 October.

To be included towards your target, the child has to have had a full course of immunization. There are 3 groups of immunizations: diphtheria/tetanus/ poliomyelitis for which the child needs 3 doses; pertussis – 3 doses; measles or mumps, measles and rubella – 1 dose.

Calculating the payment

If you give the final injection to complete a course of immunization, the child will count towards your target. If your community clinic does the 1st and 2nd, and you give the last one, you will get paid for it. The other way round and you do not. If the child has just registered with you and the final dose was given by the child's previous doctor, you will get paid for it. If the clinic does all except the final polio, and you do that, you get the payment.

Method of calculation

First you find out the number of children aged 2 on the 1st day of the quarter – (N). This is then multiplied by 3, for 3 completing immunizations. Divide this by 10 and multiply by either 7 or 9, depending on the target. You now have the figure for the number – (T) – of completing immunizations you need to reach the target. The equation is $T = N \times 3 \times 9/10$ for the higher target or $T = N \times 3 \times 7/10$ for the lower.

Next you go back to the children's records and find the number of completed courses – (C). If the number of completed courses C is more than T then you get paid. Next you need to know how much you get paid. Here you need to remember that you can only get paid for the proportion of the immunizations that you or the children's previous doctors have done compared to the whole number done. Each group of immunizations – (G) is dealt with separately. So $G = T/3$. The number of immunizations in each group of immunizations cannot exceed the target number for the group $(G \leq N)$. So if you need 17 immunizations to reach a group target and you have done 20, you will still only be credited with 17. You then add the number of completed immunizations done by you (GC) in each group $(GC1 + GC2 + GC3 = P)$. You then divide the total number of completed immunizations by the target number and multiply this by the maximum amount payable (MAX)

$(P/T \times MAX)$. The maximum payment available to you is calculated by dividing the number of children on your list by the number of children on the average doctor's list (in the 1990 SFA this is 22). This is then multiplied by the maximum payment available to this average doctor.

So for the higher target the formula is

$$T = N \times 3 \times 9/10$$

If $C \geq T$ then you get paid

$$G = T/3$$

$$GC1 + GC2 + GC3 = P$$

The amount you get paid $= MAX \times T/P$

There is a worked example in the Red Book.

Claims for payment

Claims should be made on form PT/TC1 and should be submitted to the FHSA no later than 4 months after the date the claim relates to.

Children aged 5 and under – pre-school boosters

This is worked out very similarly to the targets for children aged 2 and under.

Eligibility

The target population is defined as children who were born from the 2nd day of a particular quarter 6 years previously to the 1st day of the same quarter a year later. So your target populations for the quarter January– March 1991 will include all the children born from 2 January 1985 to 1 January 1986 inclusive.

The booster immunizations required are for tetanus, diphtheria and polio. The child has to have had all three. If the number of children who have completed booster immunizations is equal or greater than 90% or 70% of the target population, then you get paid. You will however only get paid for the proportion of immunizations that you have done. So if your target population is

50 children the higher target is 45. If you have done 40 and 6 were done by the local clinic, you will get 40/45 of the maximum payment available to you.

The maximum payment available to you is calculated by dividing the number of children on your list by the number of children on the average doctor's list (in the 1990 SFA this is 22). This is then multiplied by the maximum payment available to this average doctor.

Claims for payment

Claims should be made to your FHSA on form FP/TPB no later than 4 months after the date the claim relates to.

The important thing with targets is to anticipate the quarter. You must be able to work out your target population. Having done that, you must then be able to find out which of your children have had all their immunizations and which have not. You should do this perhaps 3 months before the start of a new quarter, so that you have time to chase up the children who have missed out.

Remember that immunizations will not count towards your target if they have been performed as part of general medical services or as a paid contract outside of general medical services. Work done by employed or attached staff under your direction will be counted towards the target.

You are responsible for reporting all immunizations to the appropriate health authority – this will help both you and them to maintain accurate records.

Cervical cytology

This is very similar to the targets for immunization for children. There are two levels of target, 80% and 50%. Payments will no longer be made for each individual cervical cytology test.

Eligibility

You will receive the higher target payment if on the 1st day of the quarter at least 80% of the eligible women on your list, aged 25 – 64 (21 – 60 in Scotland) have had an adequate smear during the period of 5½ years preceding the claim. Women aged 25 – 64 are defined as those born between the 2nd day of the same quarter 65 years earlier and the 1st day of the quarter 40 years later. So for the quarter January–March 1991 the target population includes those women born between 2 January 1926 and 1 January 1966. Target payments are now calculated on a partnership basis. The actual payment has further calculations. It depends on the number of eligible patients, compared with those on the list of the average GP, and the number of adequate smears taken as part of general medical services as opposed to those done at DHA or private clinics.

Women who have had hysterectomies are not included. You must notify your FHSA of the number of women in the age group who are in this category. No other women are excluded.

The maximum payment to you depends on the number of eligible women (25–64) on your list compared with the list of an average GP. In the 1990 SFA the average GP has 430 eligible women.

Calculating the payment

The maximum payment is the eligible number of women on your list divided by 430 and multiplied by the maximum sum payable to the average GP.

When only a proportion of the adequate smears has been completed this maximum payment is scaled down accordingly. If a woman has had more than 1 smear done in the last 5½ years, an adequate smear taken by a GP will take precedence over one taken by any other source.

On the last day of each quarter the FHSA will send you the number of target women on your list. Also included will be the number who have had smears and how many smears you did. If you disagree, you have 10 days to say so and a further 21 days to prove your case.

By 1994 all FHSAs should have the correct records on their computer systems and this will enable them to calculate payments based on their own information.

Until your FHSA has up to date records it can apportion tests whose origins are unclear in proportion with the known proportion of tests carried out by you for women on your list.

Your FHSA will accept until 1994 information based on your own records. These claims may be checked by your FHSA.

10 Vaccinations and Immunizations
(SFA paragraphs 27.1–5 and schedule 1) (FP73)

THIS section does not include the immunizations given to children under 5. These are covered by target payments.

This is an often ignored income generation source, particularly with reference to tetanus and polio.

The fee payable is indicated at the end of each paragraph for 1st, 2nd, 3rd and booster injections. Note that one fee is payable for each operation, so one fee for say tetanus, and also only one fee for a triple injection. But if you give a triple and a polio, you get two fees. The fees are paid at two levels, A and B. You get more for B than A, and B tends to be for injections completing a course or reinforcing a course. The amount paid can be found in the Red Book, and also in the various medical finance magazines.

Non-travellers

Most of the immunizations mentioned below are for groups of people at special risk who can be immunized and the immunization claimed.

1 **Diphtheria and tetanus.** A fee is payable for children aged 6 and over. Also for hospital staff at risk (A,A,B and reinforcing dose B).

2 **Tetanus.** If not already immunized – children 15–19 or on leaving school (A,A,B). If previously immunized a reinforcing dose if the patient has not had a reinforcing dose in the previous 5 years, and then the previous 5–15 years (B).

3 **Poliomyelitis.** People aged 6 and under 40 and parents or guardians of children being given oral polio. Groups at special risk (e.g. GPs, ambulance staff, nurses, laboratory staff) (A,A,B). Reinforcing doses in immunized people (aged 6 and over) entering or leaving school or entering higher education or starting work (B).

4 **Measles, mumps and rubella (MMR combined vaccine).** Children from 6–15 who have not had MMR. This should be given in preference to just measles whether or not they have had mild measles, mumps or rubella (B).

5 **Measles (single antigen).** As for 4 if they have not been immunized against or had measles (B).

6 **Rubella.** Girls aged 10–14 who have not had MMR, sero-negative non-pregnant women of child bearing age, and sero-negative men working in ante-natal clinics (B). (Have you had yours?)

7 **Anthrax.** This is for people at special risk mostly working in factories dealing the animal remains such as glue factories, tanneries and wool mills (A,A,A,B, with an *annual* reinforcement B).

Typhoid, paratyphoid, rabies, smallpox and infectious hepatitis are also payable mostly to high-risk people.

Patients travelling abroad

Apart from the groups already mentioned, payments can be claimed for people going to infected areas, or countries where a certificate is a condition of entry. The definition of Europe includes Turkey and Cyprus. Northern Europe includes Norway, Sweden, Denmark, Belgium, the Netherlands and Iceland.

1 **Typhoid and paratyphoid.** Payable by your FHSA for anyone going abroad except to Canada, USA, Australia, New Zealand and northern Europe (A,A,B).

2 **Cholera.** Travellers to Africa or Asia. *Note* if they are going to Gibralta, they may take a day trip to Morocco (A,A, with reimmunization after 6 months being A,A).

3 **Poliomyelitis.** All persons travelling to countries outside Europe except Canada, USA, New Zealand and Australia.

4 **Infectious hepatitis.** Travellers abroad except to Australia, New Zealand and northern Europe to areas of poor sanitation, especially for those less resistant to disease or those staying 3 months or more (B).

11 Minor Surgery
(SFA paragraphs 42.1–6 and schedule 1) (FP/MS)

Eligibility

TO qualify for minor surgery payments you must be included on your FHSA's Minor Surgery List. To get on, you will have to apply to and demonstrate to the FHSA some competence and that you have the necessary equipment and space. Equipment and space will probably be determined by some form of medical assessor, possibly from the Local Medical Committee.

The fee will be payable to you for undertaking minor surgery for your patients or those of your partners or group members.

No more than three session payments can be made to you in any 1 quarter (each session consists of five surgical procedures). If you are a member of a group or practice this number can be increased provided the total number of payments paid in respect of any quarter does not exceed three times the number of partners.

Look in your copy of the Red Book for the procedures.

Claims

Make your claim for payment on form FP/MS. The FHSA may check the validity of claims.

12 Rural Practice Payments
(SFA paragraphs 43.1–16)

Eligibility

HAVE you ever wondered how GPs in the more rural areas live on small lists? It is done with dispensing and rural practice payments. To get these payments, you must have at least 20% of your practice's patients living in a Rural Practice Payment Area and at least 3 miles from your main surgery by the normal route.

A Rural Practice Payment Area used to be defined as every rural district, municipal borough and urban district with a population of less than 10,000. This was based on populations in 1974 (and included such places as Milton Keynes!). There is now no definition of rurality. Rural areas will be decided by the FHSA.

If there is any doubt which is your main surgery, the FHSA will decide with the LMC.

If your practice qualifies, each patient will be separately calculated in units as to how many rural payments he is worth. The deciding factors are the distance he is from your main surgery, whether you have to walk to visit him and whether the walking is difficult. For each of these the further he lives from the surgery, the more he is worth. Difficult walking is generally worth twice ordinary walking. It is defined as the doctor having to walk for more than a quarter of a mile one way over exceptionally difficult ground. This may be steep, rough or boggy ground. You can also get payments for patients who live in areas where the route to that area from your surgery is regularly blocked at certain times of the year by flooding, snow, etc. You get 3 units per patient, irrespective of how far away they live.

If you have patients who live in areas designated by the Secretary of State as special districts, you can claim for them. Special districts are areas where there can be credits for walking and special walking, but road access is also difficult. This will probably be in mountainous areas. These patients get you 4 units each. You can get distance or walking payments as well as blocked route or special district units. If you have patients in institutions such as schools or hospitals, the patients will be worth half the number of units.

Whether or not you usually qualify for rural practice payments, you can get out-of-pocket travelling expenses reimbursed. This is allowable for visiting patients in rural practice areas, when you have had to pay tolls, ferry charges, etc.

If you are single-handed and getting rural practice payments, you can get a payment for a locum. This is to cover you only when you go on postgraduate training lasting at least 1 day.

Patients not on GP's list

Temporary residents, emergency visits and patients receiving immediately necessary treatment also qualify for rural practice payments.

Inducement payments
(SFA paragraphs 45.1 – 6)

If you work in an area which is sparsely-populated, or for some other reason is unattractive, you might get inducement payments. How much you get is decided by the Secretary of State and is reviewed each year. So do not base your pension on it! You do however get your full allowance for seniority, associate and sickness payments, even if your list is less than the normal minimum of 1,200.

13 Dispensing
(SFA paragraphs 44.1 – 5) (FP34D)

THIS can generate a substantial amount of income for the practice, and be a major source of income for rural practices. It must be run properly, or the profits may not be as large as they should be.

Eligibility

There are two classifications of GPs as far as dispensing is concerned. The practice is either a dispensing practice or a non-dispensing practice. The difference is that the latter can only dispense items which are personally administered. This includes injections, sutures, mantoux tests, coils, anaesthetics, etc.

The doctor who is in a dispensing practice can dispense any drug normally allowed for his patients included on his dispensing list. Essentially, to become a dispensing doctor, you need patients who live at least 1 mile from a chemist shop and your dispensing must not make the chemist unviable. The FHSA or the BMA may be able to help you.

What you earn is set out in the Red Book. It includes the basic price of the drug, less a discount, which is to take account of the fact that if you buy drugs in bulk, you can also get discounts. There is also an on-cost allowance of about 10.5%, again, less discount and a small allowance for a container, whether or not you supply the drug in a container. Then there is the dispensing fee less discount – the more you do, the less you get for each item. You will also get an allowance in respect of value added tax (only payable to those GPs *not* registered for VAT).

Claims

To claim, you collect up all your prescription forms for the items you dispensed in 1 month. You must then send them to the Prescription Pricing Authority by the 5th day of the next month, with the claim form FP34D. In a partnership, you must send all the partnership's prescriptions in one batch, to allow for the bulk buying discount to be calculated. You can however divide up your batch into a bundle for each partner. This will allow each partner to claim his dispensing fees, allowing for a smaller dispensing discount to be subtracted. Therefore it is important that the partners share out the dispensing reasonably evenly amongst themselves.

Accounting

Payments to the suppliers of your drug stocks must be shown on your income tax return gross, as must the income. This is because the Review Body takes a sample of tax returns to calculate the expenses part of all our income. Like netting out staff salaries, if you do it, we all suffer.

Practice protocol

When you dispense for your patients, you will need to hold a supply of drugs. This will require a big outlay. Therefore it is important to control the purchase and storage of your stock very carefully. It would seem wise to have a practice agreement on what drugs you will hold; to keep the number to a minimum and this may require a practice formulary. You may also want to have one partner and one member of staff controlling the drug stock. They should know what you have and what you are likely to need before the next delivery is to be made. They should ensure that the drugs are stored properly, and that they do not become out of date. Finally, following European law on product liability, it is important that proper records including batch numbers and suppliers are maintained.

Discounts

As the government is deducting discount from the money they pay you for your dispensed drugs, you must get a discount from your suppliers. When you first start dispensing, the discounts will not be large, but as you progress, you should be able to squeeze more from them. However, be careful not to overstretch yourself financially, because money paid to the supplier will not come back to you for at least 3 months. In that time you will pay interest on any loan. You must also be sure that what you buy will not become out of date before you dispense it. It may not be sensible therefore to buy a thousand coils or a million digoxin!

Sometimes you can get a transferred discount. Say you buy tetanus and influenza vaccines from the same manufacturer. You may be limited to a certain percentage discount on the influenza vaccine but this could be offset by getting a bigger discount on the tetanus vaccine. You might be able to get more. It is always worth haggling with your supplier, particularly if you are buying large quantities.

Oxygen therapy services

The supply of oxygen and oxygen therapy equipment is an option for dispensing practices. If you decide to do this, you will need the specific agreement of the FHSA. They will need to agree not only that you can dispense oxygen, but also how many sets you can hold. The benefit is that you get a delivery fee for taking oxygen to the patient's home. Not only that, but you get a rental fee for each giving set or stand that you hold, whether or not it is out on loan to a patient.

14 Postgraduate Education Allowance

(SFA paragraphs 37.1 – 22)   (FP/PEA)

Eligibility

THIS allowance is designed to encourage GPs to keep up to date. To qualify for the allowance you need to have completed 5 days postgraduate study a year. More precisely, you must complete 25 days, reasonably spread, in the 5 years prior to the year in which you make your claim.

You must do at least two courses in each of the three areas. These are health promotion, including the promotion of healthy living and the prevention of disease, ill health and injury; disease management, including the natural history of disease and treatment and care of the side of the terminally ill; and finally service management, including providing efficient care to patients, data and record systems, use of technology, quality assurance, etc.

Qualifying courses

Some of the qualifying terms need definition. A day is 6 hours, half a day is 3 hours, one third of a day is 2 hours and one sixth of a day is 1 hour. This can be done as one block, or more than one block. A course is a period of education approved as a course by the regional adviser in England or the Postgraduate Dean in Wales. They can be organized by your local postgraduate centre, by a group of GPs, a university, or distance learning. They will need to be assigned to one of the subject areas. The courses must also have some sort of evaluation.

Organizing or teaching on a course

If you teach on an accredited course you will be considered to have attended that course for half a day. If you stay for the whole course you are credited as attending as much as the participants. If you organize a course within your practice, the regional adviser or a course organizer are likely to give you advice on how to set it up and get it approved. You are however liable to find the powers-that-be dropping in on your course, to make sure that it is actually happening.

Value for money

No longer can you get it all free. Like the railways and British Steel, postgraduate education has to be self-financing. How you spend your money is up to you, but it might be wise to make sure that, in the best Thatcherite tradition you get good value for your money. Indeed, if you are motivated and keen, you can arrange your own courses, invite other doctors, and charge them. You thus continue to kill two birds with one stone.

Section 63 continues. Before you panic, it is only for trainers on courses for training, and for trainees. If you are a trainer, you must realize that continuing education paid for under section 63 may not count towards the postgraduate education allowance.

Claims

To claim for this allowance form FP/PEA should be completed. Claims can be made at any date after the course and the allowance will be paid for the following 12 month period. Usually no new claim can be made within 12 months of the previous claim. Your FHSA will require proof of your attendance at a course.

Your FHSA may withhold payment of the allowance if they consider the course has been unreasonably repeated or the days are unreasonably spread between the years. You are not expected to claim for more than 10 days a year.

15 Training
(SFA paragraphs 38.1 – 39.3)

SINCE 1981 it has been mandatory for GPs to have undergone a period of formal training. There are two groups of doctors who can generate income from this – trainers and trainees.

The section in the Red Book concerning trainers and trainees is a long and complex one and the section below is only a guide to point you in the right direction. If you are involved in training, you must read the appropriate section in the Red Book to claim all the benefits. Trainees, as they are employees who often have to move around, are entitled to many allowances. These must be claimed. The FHSA and/or your trainer or course organizer should help you to make sure that you receive all you are entitled to.

Trainers

Becoming a trainer

Before you can become a trainer you have to gain the approval of the Regional Postgraduate Education Committee. Applications should be made direct to the Committee.

Your practice will be visited and you will be interviewed by a panel appointed by the Sub-Committee. Normally you will need to have a practice list of at least 2000 patients. If you are thought to be a suitable person in a suitable practice, you will be appointed for an initial period of 2 years. After that reappointment will be for periods of 5 years. These lengths of time can vary from district to district.

Payments

When you get your 1st trainee, you must let the FHSA know early, so that they can arrange to make the appropriate payments. A trainee will only be in general practice for 1 year, either in one practice or split into two 6-month sessions shared by two practices. The trainer's grant cannot be paid for more than 12 months for the same trainee unless an extension is given. If arrangements between a trainee and a trainer are terminated – the FHSA and Sub-Committee should be told immediately.

If your period of approval as a trainer is due to expire before your next trainee finishes, you should not take on a new trainee without reapplication and approval from the Regional General Practice Sub-Committee. Normally you can only have one trainee at a time.

Payments made to a trainer include a training grant; the trainee's pay; reimbursement of the employer's share of the trainee's National Insurance contributions; a car allowance; the cost of an extra telephone extension in the surgery; the cost of telephone rental at the trainee's residence; and the cost of the trainee joining a medical defence organization. The trainer's grant is superannuable.

If your trainee lives away from the area in which your practice is situated, he can get a daily subsistence allowance when he is on call. There is, apart from the possible training advantages, a financial benefit to be gained from having the trainee stay in your house when he is on call. You provide board and lodging for the trainee, allowing him to answer the telephone, and you or your wife cover the telephone whilst he is out. You are then entitled to charge him for the accommodation which he then has reimbursed by the FHSA. Do not forget that like all income, this is taxable and must be declared to the Inland Revenue.

Where a trainee falls ill, if the sickness is for less than a fortnight there is no change in payments, but for more than that the trainer's grant will be stopped and the trainee's pay will be reduced by the amount of statutory sick pay and the car allowance. If your trainee goes on maternity leave, intending to return, but does not come back, the FHSA may send payments to you for her from her expected re-start date. You must let the FHSA know and return the payments less any statutory maternity pay.

Undergraduate medical students

You are entitled to a payment if you assist a recognized university department of general practice by giving medical students experience in general practice. You will be paid according to the number of students involved and the time they spend in the practice.

The session will consist of at least 2½ hours. Claims should be made on form FP/UMS.

Trainees

Payments made to a trainee come via the trainer as he is the employer. Apart from pay, National Insurance contributions and a car allowance, a trainee may be entitled to other money. Where necessary the cost of a new telephone at the trainee's house, or the cost of installation and rental of a telephone extension in the trainee's bedroom. Pay to a trainee is based upon the pay in his last hospital post.

Two thirds of the trainees subscription to a defence body is reimbursable, but you as the trainee must pay the subscription first and then make an application to the trainer.

Removal expenses

You can get payments for removal costs from a hospital post to a trainee post or between two trainee posts. Before removal you should get at least three tenders for the job, and the payments are based on the lowest tender price, irrespective of which contractor you use. Some special items of furniture may not be covered. If storage of furniture is necessary, this also may be reimbursed. Insurance of your furniture in transit is reimbursable. Legal fees and fees to estate agents may also be reimbursed.

If you are going to do all your remaining trainee jobs in the same locality, and need to move house, you can get solicitor's fees, stamp duty, land registration fees, fees required to raise finance to buy the house, the cost of a survey, including an electrical wiring test and a drains test. Even if you fail in your purchase of a house, your fees may be reimbursed.

There is a provision for payment of miscellaneous fees after you have moved house. This will include a whole variety of things such as installing a television aerial, plumbing in a washing-machine, altering curtains, cleaning the property, redirection of mail, etc.

If you rent a house, similar fees may be reimbursed, but it is specifically noted in the Red Book that estate agent's fees for arranging for you to get a tenancy are illegal, and therefore not reimbursable.

When you go to look at the area in which you are hoping to do your traineeship, your travelling costs are claimable, and when you have your job, you can get back the unexpired part of a rail or bus season ticket, and there is even the possibility of getting school fees back. If you have to leave your child behind to do his exams, you may be entitled to board and lodging costs for him.

If you cannot get a house before you start, there is provision for subsistence payments, excess daily travelling costs, and also payments for visits home.

Maternity leave

Maternity pay is much the same as for any other employee, and is the same for a hospital job. Maternity leave starts not earlier than the 29th week of the pregnancy. Payment for the first 4 weeks of leave is either full pay less National Insurance benefits, or 90% full pay less flat rate maternity benefit, whichever is the best for you. For the next 2 weeks, you get either 90% pay less flat rate maternity benefit or half pay plus National Insurance benefits. After that you get half pay plus National Insurance benefits.

If you are not going to continue your traineeship, you only get 6 weeks pay, so it is worthwhile arranging to go back to your job for a while at least. You will be employed on no less favourable conditions of work. You are entitled to time off for ante-natal care. You are also entitled to all of your statutory maternity rights. If you are away on maternity leave, the time away will count towards incremental pay rises.

Examination expenses

If you are sitting a postgraduate examination, you can get travelling and subsistence costs, but not the examination fees. Claim on form GPCF3 with confirmation from your trainer.

Retainer scheme

This is a scheme if you are not in full-time employment, say if you had small children to look after, which enables you 'to keep your hand in'. You will have the opportunity to do a small amount of specially arranged paid work, attend postgraduate education sessions and receive a small retainer. You are required to work at least one half-day per month, be ready to take on sessional work up to a maximum of 1 day per week. The FHSA will reimburse a practice which uses a retainer scheme doctor for a maximum of one notional ½-day per week. Information about this scheme can be obtained from your local regional adviser.

16 Premises
(SFA paragraphs 51.1 – 60 and 53.1 – 13

YOU can create long-term savings from your own premises, but wherever you practice, you must control costs. There are in essence three types of owner of surgery premises. The partnership may own the premises, the premises may be rented or the premises may be part of a landlord's house.

You must have the agreement of the FHSA for the premises you choose. Your FHSA will advise you on this. There are a number of basic requirements for a surgery building. They must be in a reasonable condition. They must have ease of access for all your patients, including the disabled, elderly and small children. You ought to have a properly equipped treatment room and consulting room with adequate privacy for patients. There must be toilets for both staff and patients, and you ought to have a wash basin in your consulting room. There must be adequate internal waiting areas and privacy of communication in the reception area. There must be secure space for records, prescriptions, drugs, etc., adequate fire precautions and, if the premises are used for minor surgery, suitable rooms and equipment must be provided. It is most important that you do not commit yourself to premises unless you have the agreement of the FHSA.

Rates and community charge

You are entitled to reimbursement of water rates and community charge payments. Community charge and water rates may be paid in small amounts through the year, but this could be a slightly more expensive option. When you get the bill from the local council or water authority, telephone the finance department of the FHSA and ask their staff when would be the latest time in the month for you to send them a receipt so that they could pay you at the end of the same month. This is likely to be about 2 weeks before the end of the month. You can then pay all the charge at one go, so saving time, effort and the cost of sending small amounts of money several times a year. The cost that you do carry is the interest on the charge for about a fortnight. At 15%, £5000 for 2 weeks will cost £29 in interest. Remember that if you pay it in small amounts you will have small amounts of money all carrying interest for a fortnight, or for longer if you get your receipt into the FHSA late. It is also worth remembering that even for business accounts, the bank will charge for each transaction.

Rubbish collection

You can also get 100% reimbursement of rubbish collection charges, and also for collection of sharps. Again, before entering into any agreement with someone to take away used needles and scalpels, get the agreement of the FHSA.

Rent reimbursement

Eligibility

You will receive from the FHSA an amount of money to cover the rent or, if you purpose-build or substantially alter existing accommodation a cost rent or a notional rent for owner-occupiers. You will be eligible for this if your patient list is at least 100.

Reimbursements will also be reduced if a rent is received by you from an occupant of your premises.

Privately rented premises and health centres

In this situation, you must find premises which are acceptable to the FHSA. You *must* consult your FHSA in advance to ensure the premises and their use are reasonable; those used for occasional consultations will not be reimbursed. The amount of money you get to cover the rent will be either the rent that you pay, or the rent that the district valuer thinks that you ought to pay, whichever is the lower figure. Only those premises used directly for NHS purposes will be reimbursable. You will be entitled to 100% reimbursement of community charge payments on the surgery. You can also reclaim 100% of your water rates.

In health centres where you use local authority or health authority owned premises, the situation is not very different. Here there will be an agreement covering accommodation including fixtures, rates and water rates, services and perhaps staff. The service charge is for cleaning, power, repairs, furniture, telephones, etc. The charges for accommodation and rates are fully reimbursable. Staff reimbursement may be available. The service charge is not reimbursable. The agreement that you have may vary from district to district, but generally payment will be on the number of consulting suites used, and the floor area of a consulting suite including an allowance for reception and waiting areas.

You will then be asked by the FHSA for a breakdown of your charges. Normally you pay the local or health authority and claim back what you can. You can however arrange for the FHSA to pay the authority directly and deduct an appropriate amount from your income.

Practising from someone's house

Here the situation is essentially the same, except that the FHSA will only pay for the part of the house which is used as a surgery. Where a room is used both for a surgery and for private work, the FHSA will reduce the payment further. You cannot claim for a room only used occasionally for work. Where a branch surgery is part of someone's house, and there are less than 3 surgeries per week, you are not entitled to claim.

Practice-owned premises

Here the practice works from their own premises, and does not pay rent to anyone. The payments to the practice are along the same lines as before.

The amounts of money that you are entitled to for all these reimbursements is reduced if you do a lot of private work. This includes all private patients, private NHS work, work for pharmaceutical companies, etc. Private work is defined as all work that is not for the NHS, DHAs or government departments. The amount of reduction of reimbursement that you get will depend on how much income you earn from private work. Up to 10% you lose nothing. From 10%–20% you lose 10%; 20%–30% you lose 20%; etc.

Claims for payment

Remember to actually claim for the rent, water rates, etc. Apparently every FHSA has examples of GPs who do not.

Payments will be reviewed every 3 years, and the form sent to you at this time by the FHSA should be completed and returned as soon as possible.

Cost rent scheme

If you decide to build your own premises or substantially modify newly purchased or existing practice premises, you can get reimbursement, this system is called cost rent. It is potentially one of the best forms of long term savings available to you. Essentially what you do is to put up a building. You have to pay the capital, but the FHSA pays the interest. Repayment of the capital with a low cost endowment insurance is fairly cheap. Depending on your age, and the number of years over which you want to repay, it should not be expensive. A young doctor paying off £80,000 over 20 years is likely to pay less than £100 per month. The system is a bit like owning your house with the neighbour paying the mortgage. It is also possible to sell your building back to the lenders of the money, and pay them rent. This has the advantage that you do not have to find any money each month to pay back the capital. You however do not collect the rewards when you retire. The decision is yours.

Before you begin, talk to the FHSA. It is very important that prior to committing yourself to spending money, you get a written agreement from the FHSA. This agreement should confirm that the project is viable. It should outline the method of reimbursement and an assessment of how much you will receive. It should also set a target date for completion of the project and moving in. FHSAs will require estimates, plans and specifications.

It should be forbidden to start the process of building a surgery without reading the Red Book paragraphs 51.50–60 and the succeeding schedules. Spend a weekend reading it and making sure that you understand it. Failure to follow the rules can be very expensive indeed. The Red Book gives good advice. See paragraph 51.50–8. The starting point is to find a piece of land. Do not buy it at this stage. You may want to get an option to buy it, but until you ensure that you can put a surgery on it, and do not want to spend any money. You can work out the approximate amount of money you can spend on a new building by looking at the schedules at the end of paragraph 51. It also depends upon whether you are creating a new building or modifying an existing building. A new building gives you Rate A. Modification gives you Rate B. If your modification of an existing building involves substantial new building work you get a bit of each.

Next look at schedule 3. From this you get the cost rent limit band for the area in which you live. Next go to schedule 1 for the number of partners in your practice. This assumes that you can persuade the FHSA that you will, at least some of the time, all be consulting in the building at one time. Remember that a trainee does not count as a partner. You will however get extra space if you are a training practice. The calculation is then relatively simple. You take the basic practice unit, giving you an area available to you. Add to this extra space for nurses. trainees and a dispensary where appropriate. You then multiply the number of allowable square metres by the appropriate rate in the correct cost limit band.

Now you add to that amount of money an extra 15% to cover the cost of externals such as paths, parking spaces, fences, etc. You also have to pay architects, surveyors etc. They do not come cheap. You are allowed an extra 10% for them. This gives you the figure for the cost of the building, but you also may add the cost of statutory fees for planning and building regulations.

It may, at a later date, be evident that the site chosen had particular unforeseeable problems. These might be forgotten drains which need diverting, or the ground might be unstable, needing more extensive foundations.

It is probably worth getting the agreement of other interested parties for you to move into a new surgery. These would include possibly other doctors in the town, the Community Health Council and the District Council.

You now have the basis upon which to work. Your next task is to get the various professionals around you. You will need your accountant, your practice banker and solicitor, and an architect. Your solicitor will ensure that you can get the land bought at the right time. Also that you and your patients have proper access to the land.

Raising the money to create your surgery should not cause too much difficulty. Most banks and some insurance companies are now well versed in the cost rent scheme, and are happy to help you. Whether you go for a fixed rate or a variable rate loan is up to you with the advice of your accountant.

As you are dealing with large amounts of money, small variations in interest rates make a big difference. One-quarter per cent per year on £250,000 is £625, or more than £50 each month. For fixed rate loans, the rate of interest you will get from the FHSA is fixed at the rate charged for these loans by the General Practice Finance Corporation on the day that you sign the contract to build. This is important to understand. You will almost certainly sign contracts some time before you fix the rate from your money lender. So if interest rates are rising, the shorter time between signing contracts and fixing the amount you pay, the better. The opposite is true for falling rates. For example, the rates may be going up ½% every second month. If you fix the FHSA rate at 10% and then do not set the payment rate for 4 months, you will be paying 11% out. In this case you might be better off with a variable rate at the beginning. If the rates are falling by ½% per month, the same delay would earn you 1%.

It is very important to be clear about the terms of a loan. Can you repay the loan early? – usually at a cost. What happens when a partner retires? – will they lend to an incoming partner? When is the interest rate on a fixed rate loan fixed? – probably when you take your first instalment.

Finding an architect can be difficult. It is very like finding a doctor, and what you end up with, may be good, bad or not very interested in you. It is worth spending time and effort on the right choice. The Royal Institute of British Architects will give you a list of their members. This list may not be very selective. You need someone who knows about surgeries. It may be that you know another doctor who has built a surgery and can help. The FHSA may well be able to help you. Be careful about your choice. When you have found your architect, begin with an understanding of what you are doing and what you want them to do. Think about the possibility of a relationship based on a written contract. This has the advantage of making everything clear, but it can be limiting. The architect will start by providing you with some sketch plans. Do not be bullied into accepting an outline until you have what you want. Do not forget your staff. They are likely to have ideas at least as good as yours. They will also know what sort of reception area they will need.

There are some basic necessities which ought to be considered. Can you get an ambulance close to the building? Can you get a stretcher down the corridor? Are there enough seats in the waiting area? Can you go from your consulting room to the toilet without going through the waiting room? What about vandal-proofing the building? There are many possibilities to think about. You will get many ideas from visiting other surgeries, especially new ones.

Once you have agreed an outline, detailed plans start to appear. Ensure that these fit what you want. It is probably worth spending an afternoon with someone from the architects' office to go through the detailed plans. This will guarantee that you understand what you are getting. You will know which way the doors hinge. Where you will be sitting, either with a fixed desk of a freestanding one. It is important that you get it right, as all the wall plugs could be out of reach if you do not!

When tenders go out, you may have an interest in who is invited to tender. A talk with the architect will sort out firms who are able to do the work. There may be tendering for work other than the main contractors. Steel erectors, electricians, heating engineers, etc., may be chosen. Again, you might have an interest in who gets the jobs. It is your money which pays them.

When the work starts, it is worthwhile having one partner with whom the architect can liaise, so that decisions can be made quickly. That partner should be able to visit the site most days to make sure that things are proceeding as planned and go to site meetings. It is at these meetings that you will discover the problems being encountered. You might be able to solve some of them. Do not forget to let your patients know what is going on.

The day you move in is important. Not only are you, your staff and your patients finding your way around, but this is the day when payments from the FHSA start.

For the first few months you will be paid on an estimate of your final cost rent. This is the interim cost rent. It takes some time for the FHSA to calculate the final cost rent. They have to check that the building comes up to standard. Also that moveable items such as loose furniture, loose carpets (that is, not fitted) are not included in the cost rent. They will need to find out how much interest was payable to the money lender whilst the building was being constructed. This interest will be rolled-up or aggregated by the lender and added to the capital sum to be repaid. It is also allowable against the cost rent.

Every 3 years after moving in, you will have an opportunity to have your building revalued for cost rent purposes. This is so that as building values rise, you can maintain an economic rent. Initially the value of the building will be less than the amount of money you have spent. The cause of this is the rolled-up interest. After 6, or more likely 9 years, the value of your building will have risen above the cost to you. The problem is that the valuation is done by the district valuer, who tends to give conservative values. It is his valuation upon which the FHSA will pay for the next 3 years at least. You can appeal against his valuation.

If your building cost £250,000 to construct and another £50,000 in interest, its initial value will still be £250,000. Say building values rise 5% per year. At 3 years your building will be worth £289,000. At 6 years £335,000. At this point you get the building valued yourself so that you understand its worth. Assuming that the value is correct, you ask the FHSA to value your building. Again assuming that the district valuer comes to the same conclusion, the FHSA will pay your cost rent at the same interest rate as before, but based on a new value. What you do with the extra money coming in is up to you.

The last thing to do is to get your solicitor to bring your practice agreement up to date. You now have a very large asset which needs protecting in case there is trouble sometime in the future.

When you retire, you sell your share of the building back to the remaining partners. You will probably have repaid the original loan. As a consequence, you may well have in excess of £100,000 to add to superannuation lump sum. The practice can either keep your returned share of the building for themselves or sell it to an incoming partner. The newcomer will be able to arrange a loan as you did.

With this system, everybody is happy. You have a solid pension scheme, that is difficult to better. You and your staff have good working conditions. The patients have a well-presented and adequate medical centre. The government can boast of how well it has provided for primary health care needs.

Remember that for a cost rent scheme to work and be completed successfully your FHSA must be kept informed of every development and detail.

17 Improvement Grants
(SFA paragraphs 56.1–18 and schedules 1, 2)

THIS is a scheme to help doctors who own or have a long-term lease on their building. It is to enable the practice to improve the surgery. You will need to have a surgery with consulting rooms and waiting room, etc., and the surgery must already be eligible for reimbursement of rent and rates. The grant is for the provision of new rooms, improved toilet facilities, better wheelchair access, hand wash basins in consulting rooms, double glazing, pram parks and so on. Improvement grants are not for you to buy land to build on, or for replacement of old buildings. You cannot replace furniture or repair structural damage either. Where you are adding to a building, you must have at least a covered corridor joining the old to the new. The size of the finished building must not exceed the dimensions laid out for cost rent purposes (paragraph 51, schedule 1).

If you decide to apply for a grant, you will need a professionally estimated cost, sketch plans of what you have now and what you hope to have, and a schedule of work. You will also need a note from the local council that they have no objection. Finally, if the surgery is rented, you need written permission from your landlord. If you do not have all of these, you will get no further.

If you get the go-ahead, you will be told how much of the grant will need to be repaid and when. If you get agreement, you will be offered between one third and two thirds of the total cost. The maximum amount that you can get is set out in schedule 2. You will get this money after the project is complete. The sting comes in paragraph 56.16, which tells you that you cannot set the cost of any of the work for which an improvement grant has been paid against tax.

18 Employing Staff
(SFA paragraphs 52.1–33) (PS 1, 2, 3, 4)

THIS is one of the areas which has potentially changed a great deal with the introduction of the new contract.

The basis of employing people to help you is no different to that for any small business. They have all the rights and responsibilities of any employee. In addition, you are responsible for their actions whilst they are at work. If a receptionist refuses a request for a visit or turns away a patient who comes to the reception desk, it is as if you yourself had done it. Consequently you must take great care when you appoint someone to your staff. At interview you must make clear the standards required of surgery staff. The primary requirement is that all information in the surgery is confidential to the patient concerned. There are also some special problems to be encountered in general practice. There are dangers from disease-carrying sharps, dressings, etc. Drugs are around, they must treat them with respect. This is true both for drugs handled and also for drugs prescribed.

There is clear advantage in writing all these and similar problems down in the employees' contracts of employment. You have a legal requirement to provide your employees a contract of employment within 13 weeks of them starting work. Failure of your staff to do their job properly is quite likely to cost you money. If that happens and you sack them without going through the correct dismissal procedures it will cost you even more. If you are taken to an industrial tribunal and effectively fined, the fine is not reimbursable. You must have someone in the practice who understands current employment legislation.

Practice Staff Scheme

Under the Practice Staff Scheme, the FHSA has the facility to reimburse you in part or wholly for the costs of employing staff. Staff employed on 1 April 1990 when the new contract came in will continue to have their pay reimbursed at 70%. This was guaranteed by the Government. They have not guaranteed to reimburse any pay increases or increases in salary caused by a change in job description.

Under this new scheme you can claim for a wider range of staff than previously, for example physiotherapists, chiropodists, counsellors, etc.

Reimbursement of your staff pay at the moment will normally be 70% of their salary plus 100% of their National Insurance contributions. The balance is supposed to be repaid to you in the expenses part of your income. That is dependent upon everyone filling in their tax returns accurately and not netting out income and expenditure. However, the situation for new staff is that you will have to apply for reimbursement for their salary, National Insurance contributions, training costs, agency costs, holiday and sick leave and so on. Each of these may or may not be directly reimbursed. If they are reimbursed, the rate of reimbursement can be anything from 0 to 100%

If you decide to allow your staff a pay increase, the FHSA are allowed to let you have a proportion of the increases back. They can also decide the date from which a rise is reimbursable and what qualifications are required of your staff for reimbursement of their pay.

Any decision made by the FHSA will last for at least 3 years. They have the right to decide how much longer, if any, the agreement to reimburse will last.

These regulations make for a very delicate decision to be made when you take someone on. Would you be better with a fixed-term contract of employment, after which the employee would be eligible for consideration as to whether they would get a new contract? This is rather like the situation in professional football where players at the end of their contracts worry about being re-employed, or if they are good, moving to another club offering better terms of employment. Could we have the introduction of transfer fees for receptionists? When will we have the first £1,000,000 receptionist? The problem is that a good receptionist takes years to train. It might be the case that you should bite the bullet and offer unlimited contracts, with increasing benefits for long service. These benefits could include increasing holidays, pensions and perhaps a lump sum after each decade. What you do and how you do it is up to you.

There is a facility in the regulations for you to have advances on the amount to be reimbursed. In this, you will get 30% of the previous quarter's claim paid at the end of each month of a quarter. The balance should be paid at the end of the first month of the next quarter along with the first payment of the new quarter.

If you work in a health centre with local authority employed ancillary staff, the situation is not very different. You will pay the health authority the amount due to them for staff pay and claim it back from the FHSA.

You must know exactly what can be claimed for, how it can be justified and which forms are required. If you do not take into account the changes in practice staff claims you could lose money and reduce your ability to run your practice efficiently.

19 Computer Costs
(SFA paragraphs 58.1–22)   (CM 1, 2, 3, 4)

IF you get yourself a new computer, you can get some of the cost reimbursed. This includes bought or leased machines and whether or not you are upgrading from an old one. The reimbursement is for the cost of the machine, the cost of maintaining the machine and the information on it and also for the cost of staff to load the information onto the machine.

The amount reimbursed, for the full cost of system purchase and installation, is up to half of the amount that you pay. It is dependent upon the FHSA having the funds available and the scheme will only last until 31 March 1991. Valid claims which are not considered in one financial year can be resubmitted the following year. There is a 50% reimbursement for leasing costs but this is on a sliding scale based on practice size.

Staff costs incurred in setting up the computer system can be reimbursed up to 70% of the actual costs. However, do not buy a computer solely on the basis of getting your money back, because you might not. As with all projects, if you have any doubt, having read the Red Book, ask the FHSA.

Remember that because this payment is cash-limited the FHSA can take into account the effects of computerization on patient care and administrative efficiency, when considering your claim.

20   Sickness and Maternity Payments
(SFA paragraphs 48.1 – 32)

IF you fall ill, you may be able to claim payments from the FHSA to help with paying a locum. Whether or not you can get the money depends upon the average number of patients each remaining partner is left with. A single-handed doctor will almost certainly be allowed the payment – that is unless he works in a group. Payment also depends upon how long you are ill. For less than 2 weeks, a full-time partner away will need to leave the partners with at least 3,600 patients each. Between 2 and 6 weeks, it is 3,100 each, and over 6 weeks, 2,700. So if you have a partnership of 4 and 10,000 patients, a partner away ill will leave the remaining partners with an average of 3,333 each. His illness will need to last at least 2 weeks to qualify.

How long the payment lasts depends on how long the sick doctor has been a principal, a trainee in general practice, in the forces or civil service, etc., qualifying for the NHS Superannuation Scheme. If he has 5 years service, he will get 6 months of full payment and 6 months of half payment. With less than 5 years service, the payments are scaled down.

There are exceptions to the requirements. These are at the discretion of the FHSA. This covers situations where there is a large area to cover, the remaining doctors are elderly or unwell themselves. If you think that you might qualify on these grounds, speak to the FHSA.

If the cause of the doctor being away is an accident for which he can get damages, the FHSA will not pay for a locum. They may however make an advance until damages are collected. The FHSA will need medical certification that the doctor is not fit to work.

If one of your partners falls ill, tell the FHSA. They will be able to calculate whether you are eligible for payment. If you are, then get a sick note from your ill partner and send it to the FHSA. If you do not qualify, but are finding life difficult, explain your problem to the FHSA as they might be able to offer you some sort of assistance.

Maternity payments

Maternity payments are similar to sickness payments. There are however some differences. First of all, they are only available to women. Secondly there is no list size criteria. You will need to write to the FHSA stating that you intend to return to practice after the baby is born. Payments continue for 13 weeks. This period of time can be taken before and after the child's birth depending on how you wish to divide it. If you are away for more than 13 weeks because of illness you may qualify under the sickness provisions.

21 The Practice Accountant

YOUR accountant is a very important member of your income generation team. This fact has three major consequences on your relationship with the accountant.

Most practices already have an accountant, but if you do not have one, you must choose yours with care. You must ensure that the accountant understands the particular ways in which you are paid, and also the importance of presenting the accounts in the correct manner. This is because the Review Body looks at a percentage of accounts presented to the Inland Revenue to estimate the expenses part of the award for the next year.

Your accountant's fees will pay for themselves if he is doing his work properly. You will probably be increasing your income by using his skills. You must ensure that his work is done at least to your satisfaction.

Finally and most importantly, do not keep things from him. Doing that could result in disaster for both of you, but will probably end in you losing money and your accountant.

Your accountant will provide a number of services for you. Some of these services can be done by you or your staff, and if necessary checked by the accountant. These services are:

1 Receive statements of income from partners (or in some cases a random bundle of receipts) from approximately the last partnership year.
2 Balance your books, ensuring that all money paid to the practice has been lodged properly in the correct account. Also that all payments made by the practice have been made from the correct account.
3 Ensure that your bank statements correspond to your money movements.
4 Audit your accounts, although this is not done by many practices.
5 Prepare your accounts.
6 Ensure that each partner receives the correct amount of drawings from the practice.

7   Provide you with advice on money management, so that you make the most of the money in your accounts, and make sure that your tax bill is no larger than it ought to be.

8   Provide you with an informed contact with the tax man.

9   Ensure that in any large financial undertaking such as a cost rent building, you have the necessary flow of money and do not get into any big money or cash flow troubles. He will also make sure that you get the best deal from the various financial institutions.

Your accountant is someone who should be seen as part of the primary health care team. Most of the good things we do are paid for, either directly or indirectly. Moreover many of the other members of the primary health care team do things which can earn you money, or allow you to earn money.

Like other members of the primary health care team, the accountant needs to be educated by you in the ways of general practice. He needs to know how you earn money, how you employ people, how you can have several sidelines – private patients, dispensing, factory jobs, etc. He must have a copy of the statement of fees and allowances.

Your practice may have a turnover of £500,000 or more, making it a good-sized business by any standards. This sort of turnover needs to be controlled and checked very carefully. Your accountant will do this. He will however provide you with the figures and the direction for you to do the controlling from day to day. He is expensive, and it is important not to waste his time. He will probably want to reconcile the cheques going out with the invoices, and the income with the FHSA vouchers and the paying-in book. To present him with a cheque book, a paying-in book, and a cardboard box full of various pieces of paper, will cause his heart to sink and his bill to rise. So, as invoices are received, store them chronologically with a note as to when they were paid and how they were paid – petty cash or cheque. If they were paid by cheque record the cheque number. It may be easier to mount the invoices on a piece of paper, write the details on the paper, and store it in a ring-binder or lever-arch file. You can divide the stored invoices into monthly sections with card dividers. Cheque books and paying-in books can be numbered as you receive them from the bank, so that they also can be kept in chronological order.

Whilst the cheque book is being used, the covers are retained, but when the cheque book is empty and all the cheques have been cleared by the bank, tear the covers off, saving only the bit over the cheque stubs. This will save you or your accountant searching through cheque books unnecessarily.

The accountant may want to come to your surgery to write the books up, and to reconcile income and expenditure. This will save you taking or sending all the books to him, perhaps forgetting one or two and thereby taking more time and adding to his bill.

It will be worthwhile talking to your accountant about any major change in the practice, or indeed in your personal life. You may decide to buy a new car. Does your accountant have any opinions on when to buy, how to finance it, or even how much to spend? You need a new ECG – he may be able to get you a good deal to finance it, or know someone who can. If a new surgery is planned, he will be able to tell you of the financial consequences.

Occasionally there will be times when he will make a suggestion to improve your financial standing with the bank or with the Inland Revenue. A practice with a turnover of £600,000 a year, will move £50,000 a month. So some of the time you will be in credit with the bank, and sometimes you will owe money to the bank. Where the best place to have the balancing point is a question best answered by the accountant.

The date of your financial year-end is important. Again your accountant will tell you when is the best time. He will if necessary change it for you. The reason that the date of your year-end is important is based on the fact that as a self-employed person you pay your tax on the profits of the previous year. Accountants call this 'the preceding year basis'. That is the profits declared at the end of the financial year within the last fiscal year. The fiscal year goes from 6 April to 5 April.

If your practice financial year ended on 31 March 1989, the profits declared were in the fiscal year 6 April 1988 to 5 April 1989. You will pay the tax on those profits the next year – that is 1989/90. If, however, your financial year ended on 30 April 1989, that was in the fiscal year 6 April 1989 to 5 April 1990 and tax on the profits will not be payable until the year 1990/91. So in effect you pay tax not 1 but 2 years later.

This has two effects. If you move your practice financial year to 30 April from 31 March you permanently delay paying tax on 11 months profits. You also, if your profits rise each year, make a continual saving. So if you have a financial year ending early in the fiscal year, you can nearly double the tax savings.

Someone starting out in an established practice gets in effect a tax holiday. This is because he has left a PAYE system, being taxed on current earnings to start schedule E where he is taxed on the previous year. In this instance, he has already paid tax on the previous year and so there is no preceding year to be taxed on. This is a useful help for a hard-pressed junior partner. He must remember however that the next year, he will have a previous year for tax, and his monthly cheque will go down suddenly as his tax is taken off.

Practice accounts

The minimum requirement for these is that they be signed by an accountant as being accurate. In most practices the accountant will prepare them as well. Practice accounts serve several purposes. They provide the partners with a statement of how much they have earned and how the profits were shared. They also give information on how much, and where they have spent money, highlighting areas of strength and weakness. They allow you to compare your performance in 1 year with the year before. They allow some forecasting on future profits. Finally they provide the Inland Revenue with a basis upon which to form your tax demand for the next year. They are not always easy to read and understand, but with a bit of patience they can be mastered.

Drs McDonald & Tudor
Financial Account for the period
1 May 1990 to 30 April 1991   A

Contents

1. Accountants Certificate
2. Trading Profit and Loss Account
3. Balance Sheet and Schedule of Fixed Assets
4. Partnership Capital Accounts

Accountants Certificate   B

In accordance with instructions given to us we have prepared, without carrying out an audit, the Trading Profit and Loss Account and Balance Sheet from your accounting records and from information and explanations given to us.

Keegan Waddle & Beardsley
Chartered Accountants
Gallowgate Chambers
Strawberry Lane
Newcastle upon Tyne NE6 SUO

Drs McDonald & Tudor
Trading Profit and Loss Account for the Year Ended
30 April 1991

C

		1991		1990	
		£	£	£	£
General Medical Services			97,522		76,931
Premises	D		15,360		1,528
Ancillary Help			29,318		22,366
Sundry Fees			11,013		8,376
Hospital Fees			226		510
Deposit Account Interest (net)			477		145
Sickness Benefit			158		1,324
			154,074		111,180

Less Overheads

Salaries and National					
Insurance		40,587		30,500	
Pension Scheme					
Contributions		3,441		3,148	
Locum Fees	E	36		2,552	
Medical Consumables		1,025		676	
Repairs and Renewals	F	615		61	
Telephone Charges		1,658		1,061	
Printing, Postage and					
Stationery		2,455		853	
Cleaning and Canteen	F	1,155		–	
Sundry Expenses		2,473		1,315	
Heating and Lighting	F	1,158		–	
Health Centre Charges	G	4,599		3,859	
Insurance		550		172	
Branch Surgery		140		280	
Loan Interest	H	18,313		–	
Hire Purchase Interest		211		13	
Bank Interest and Charges		1,409		693	
Equipment Leasing	F	1,361		202	
Accountancy Charges		896		630	
Depreciation –					
Fixtures and Fittings		755		451	
			82,837		46,466

NET PROFIT FOR THE PERIOD			71,237		64,714

DIVIDED AS FOLLOWS:

Dr M. McDonald			35,619		38,828
Dr J. Tudor	I	35,618		25,886	
			71,237		64,714

Drs McDonald and Tudor
Balance Sheet as at 30 April 1991

		30 April 1991 £	£	30 April 1990 £	£
FIXED ASSETS	J		135,875		4,090
CURRENT ASSETS					
New Premises Suspense Account	K	–		59,859	
Sundry Debtors and Prepayments		8,108		1,610	
Bank Accounts		5,596		5,687	
		13,704		67,156	
CURRENT LIABILITIES					
Bank Account Current Account		2,007		–	
Sundry Creditors and Accruals		718		1,057	
Hire Purchase Creditors		1,082		1,771	
Bank Loan	L	4,612		185	
Equipment Fund		1,548		512	
New Premises Loan	M	132,534		59,770	
		142,501		63,295	
NET CURRENT (LIABILITIES)/ASSETS			(128,797)		3,861
			(1,390)		7,955

REPRESENTED BY

PARTNERSHIP CAPITAL ACOUNTS
Dr M. McDonald   £3,292
Dr J. Tudor   £3,786
                      £7,078

Drs McDonald and Tudor
Schedule of Partnership Capital Accounts for the Period N

1 May 1990 to 30 April 1991

	McDonald £	Tudor £	Total £
Opening Capital	4,277	3,419	7,695
Share of Profit	35,619	35,618	71,237
	39,896	39,037	78,932
Less			
Drawings O	36,604	35,251	71,855
Closing Capital	3,292	3,786	7,077

Notes on the practice accounts

A   This will normally be a year. There will be occasions when it may be longer or shorter. This might be caused by a change in partnership, or perhaps a change in practice accounting year.

B   This is your guarantee. It also outlines exactly what has been done by the accountant.

C   Accounts should normally allow you to compare the period of account with the previous period.

D   In this period of account, the practice completed new premises and moved into them. The income therefore includes a big increase in payments from the FHSA for premises.

E   There was a partner away ill. He was replaced by a locum, for which an insurance company paid.

F   These are all increased because of the move into their own premises. Cleaning and electricity were previously included in health centre charges.

G   Health centre charges were carried forward from the previous year.

H   Loan interest was accumulated whilst the surgery was under construction. This will be rolled into the total borrowing from the lender. It will then be allowable under the cost rent regulations.

I   John Tudor reached parity in this year.

J   The fixed assets are now mainly the new surgery building.

K   A suspense account in needed to pay the builders before money comes from your long-term money lender. It is short-term borrowing and may well come from the practice banker.

L   A bank loan may be needed to finance items to go inside your new surgery. These might include wastebins, table-lamps, chairs, crockery or even a new computer.

M   This is the main loan for the building.

N   Capital accounts allow for exact reckoning at the end of a year, after the drawings have been based on your accountant's guesswork on what you ought to be drawing.

O   Drawings include not only your cheque at the end of the month, but also your tax liability and superannuation. It might also involve endowment insurance premiums for the surgery loan.

There are some points specific to general practice with which an accountant, not used to dealing with your affairs, may not be aware of. It is important that he understands that the money received by the practice has had superannuation taken from it. The superannuation is part of your income, and if one of your partners has opted out of the NHS superannuation scheme, it will make a big difference to his drawings.

The Review Body and your accounts

A selection of tax returns are taken by the Review Body to calculate the expense part of all doctors remuneration. Your accountant must separate in his accounts for the Inland Revenue the money paid to ancillary staff, and the reimbursed part of that money. He must not subtract one from the other, entering it as a single expenditure item (a process known as netting-out). If your accounts are used, and you have netted-out accounts, it will be assumed that the netted-out figure is the gross expenditure figure. The result will be that the average for all GPs expenditure will be lower. Consequently the expenses part of your income and that of every GP in the country (including mine!) will be lower.

Net profit percentage

Net profit percentage can be a measure of how well you are doing. It is calculated by the equation:

$$\text{Net profit \%} = \text{Profit/turnover} \times 100$$

It shows how much of your practice turnover you are taking home. Generally you are looking for about 25–30%. If you are significantly below, you may not be earning much at all – you may already be in financial trouble. The suggestion is that you may have too high an expenditure level, and you will need to look at your outgoings. It could indicate to the Inland Revenue you are claiming excessive expenditure. Indeed, if you are significantly outside the averages for most practices, he is liable to look very carefully at your practice to see whether your tax returns are true.

A very high percentage may indicate that you are underinvesting. In this case a selective increase of your spending in the practice (perhaps in practice nurses, equipment allowing you to earn in new areas, or a coat of paint to make the surgery less daunting for your patients) will increase your turnover, and with it your profit.

Outgoings

You will have outgoings which can be entered in either your personal or practice accounts. It may be best to put most expenses through the practice account. There are two reasons for this. Firstly practice accounts are easier to arrange in a tax-efficient way. Practice borrowing in a loan account may be tax deductible. Secondly you may, for example, need a video camera to record your trainee's consultations. If the camera is purchased by the practice, it may be easier to demonstrate to the Inland Revenue that you are going to use it solely and exclusively for your business than if you bought it yourself. Remember that for most items to be tax allowable, they must be for the sole and exclusive use of your practice.

22 Non-National Health Service Work

Private patients

THE problems encountered here seem to fall into three categories.

1 Charging the right amount.
2 Getting your money after you have done the work.
3 Separating private from NHS work.

Charging will generally need to be on a basis of how much work you have done for the patient. Generally fees are based on a charge for a consultation. Visits, night and weekend work would be worth more. It is suggested that you charge what the market will bear. In some areas patients will be prepared to pay more than elsewhere. The difficulty is that if you overcharge, patients will not come back to you, and you could lose out on recommendations for new patients. If you are not skilled in judging the market, start low and work up. Some charges are preset. These would include laboratory and X-ray charges, where the suppliers will have fees set down that you can pass on to your patient. You can add an arrangement fee, that is up to you.

Getting the cash out of your patient seems to cause more problems. A good receptionist and a Visa account seem to be the most effective way. Once the patient is out of your surgery, life becomes more difficult. Sending your patient an invoice is the way to start, but what you do after that depends on how much you are owed, and how much you want the money. It is probably worth writing once or twice more. If he will still not pay, your best recourse is to the small claims court. This is not expensive, and can be effective. It is however, time-consuming. Sending in the bailiffs does not do a lot for your public image. You may decide to put it all down to experience and hope he comes back for more treatment, when you can charge him before you begin.

Where services are charged to you for you to reclaim from the patient, as may be done from some hospital departments, it may be wise to get the money from your patient before he goes.

One of the most common reasons for doctors to be invited to FHSA service committee hearings or even Hallam Street is their confusion of private and NHS work. If your patient is registered with your practice you must not under *any* circumstances charge him for work covered by the NHS. There are however services not covered by the NHS, such as certificates for insurance companies, letters for rehousing and against jury service, medicals for employers and the various driving licences. If you are in doubt, ask your FHSA, but my advice is to err on the side of not charging. Not charging in times of doubt will cost you a few pounds only. Charging when you should not have done, can lead to months of trouble with an expensive end.

When you send your patients to the hospital for investigations for non-NHS reasons, you must tell the hospital. Failure to do so might end up with you having to pay the charge out of your own pocket. Hospital auditors are starting to look out for this so tell and pay up, then charge your patient.

Private medicals

These can be a regular source of income. There are several reasons for people to want a private medical:

- Heavy Goods Vehicle and Public Service Vehicle licences both require a full medical before the driving test can be taken. They are also needed annually for drivers of these vehicles after the age of 65.
- Insurance companies require medicals done before providing insurance cover.
- Some countries require medical evidence of fitness before they will allow immigration.
- Many sports such as diving and boxing ask that a competitor can demonstrate his fitness to partake.
- Adoption societies also require that potential adoptive parents show that they are fit and healthy.

All of these categories will, if you wish, pay for a medical. Many of the people coming will be your own patients.

However, it pays to let organizing bodies know that you are able and available to do these medicals. Why not write to each insurance company with whom you have any dealings to say that you are there and can do any medicals that they may require. You will need to include what times of the day you can do them, how appointments are made and how extensively you are prepared to go. For instance, are you going to take blood samples for HIV testing? Have you got an ECG or a spirometer? Local taxi firms and haulage companies are more likely to come to you for their medicals if they know about you. You must be *very* careful not to overstep the GMC guidelines on advertising.

Most of these medicals are easy to do, they are just time-consuming. Start at the top of the form, asking the questions of the patient as stated on the form. Then do the examination, including all that is asked of you. If the form states that a tooth count is wanted, then provide them with an accurate tooth count, they are paying. Insurance companies are generally reliable payers.

One problem encountered is when examining your own patients. If you find something which would stop him doing the activity that he wants to do, or would raise his insurance premium, there may be a temptation to overlook it. Avoid this. You are acting at this time for the insurance company of whomever. You will maintain your professional integrity, and may be asked to do further work. For some medicals such as for sport, by not cheating, you will not be putting your patient at risk. A patient dying underwater when you have just passed him fit to aqualung does not enhance your reputation.

Lawyers are also a source of income. They need reports on patients – usually to help them in a damages claim or to keep them out of gaol. Charge a proper amount for your work, perhaps remembering how much a solicitor will charge you when you buy a house! If you are asked to attend court, write to the solicitor to tell him your hourly rate. He cannot then reasonably dispute the size of your bill.

Occupational medicine

Being a doctor to a local employer is a common and enjoyable way of adding to your finances. For some practices, it is a major source of income. Before getting in too deep, remember that if you earn more than 10% of your total income from non-NHS or government sources, you may find your staff and accommodation reimbursement being reduced.

When a new factory or business sets up, the owners may need a medical adviser. There is no reason for you not to approach them, and offer your services. They may need someone with specialist knowledge. If you have that, you will be extremely useful, if not, you might still be able to provide some cover, perhaps examining their new recruits. Most things are within common medical knowledge, and those that are not can be learnt. Sometimes you will need help from a university department of occupational medicine. This will be most likely when the company is working with specialist chemicals which need to be monitored. The university will be able to tell you what to look out for.

An employer most often needs someone to make sure that people just recruited are fit for employment and to record any defects. You will need to look around the workplace to see the hazards for yourself, so that you carry out the most relevant examinations. If the work is heavy, you may want to concentrate on weight-bearing joints. If it is noisy, an audiogram is essential.

Where you do the medicals is up to you and the employer. There may be a medical room, which has the advantage that no one is away from work for very long, but it may be noisy. The employer may prefer for you to do the work in your surgery, providing all the equipment. If they want you to do regular examinations of all their staff, you will probably need to go there. This is also true if you are going to do long sessions, or if the factory is a long way from your surgery.

Most employers seem most keen to get a clear answer to their questions. For instance:

- Is this man fit to be employed? – Yes, no, or yes within clear boundaries.
- Can this man be retired on ill health grounds within the terms of the company insurance? – Yes or no, and why.
- How long is he going to be away from work? – 2 weeks, 2 months, he will never be back.
- What to expect when he does get back? – He should be away no more than anyone else, he will be likely to have more episodes of back pain.

Make your opinion clear.

How much you charge is up to you. There is a scale of charges suggested by the British Medical Association, but you do not have to abide by that. The method of charging is up to you. You may decide on a fixed fee – so much per month. You could charge an amount for each examination. You can adopt part of each system, with a smallish retainer and a fee for each bit of work done. It depends on what you agree with the employer.

Government departments

The government has many needs for doctors. The armed forces need civilian doctors to examine recruits. The prison service cannot provide full cover with its full-time medical staff. The vast majority of medicals for attendance allowance and mobility allowance are done by ordinary GPs. The police need GPs as police surgeons to examine not only their officers, but also prisoners. There is an increasing demand here for female doctors to examine victims of assault. The demand from government is huge and increasing. If you are interested, write to the powers-that-be and offer your services.

Some work for these sections of government require specific training, but they may provide this. Most, however, is no more complicated than any other medical work. Generally they will set down parameters within which the medical must be performed. Payment from government departments is not negotiable, but is generally not too bad. They tend to be reasonably prompt payers. They will also pay arrears after a pay rise.

23 Petty Cash

THERE is a small but steady flow of petty cash through most practices. Control of this is very important. Most doctors will know of the type of work which earns a few pounds at a time, and often as cash. This includes private sick notes, cremation fees, some medicals, the occasional immunization certificate and so on. It is very easy to lose track of this income, but the Inland Revenue will be aware of it. Small indiscretions they will overlook, but they will maintain full records. If however you get into a major investigation, they can go back 7 years to find if you have erred from the straight and narrow. If they find that you have not been 100% accurate, they can go back another 7 years. They can do it over and over again. It is therefore foolish not to do the job accurately and with care. You have enough burdens without having the Inland Revenue investigating you.

The maintenance of an efficient and well-regulated petty cash system, control and regulation should be integral part of any practices bookkeeping arrangements.

Similarly many of your practice expenses are most easily and cheaply paid in cash. Things such as lightbulbs, perhaps the gardener or the milkman. Many of these sort of things are most appropriately left to a trusted member of staff. This may be a practice manager. She will need to keep an accurate record of where and when the money has gone. She will need to get receipts. The record should be kept in a cash book. Here she will record when she received money from the practice current account and the cheque number. Each payment item will need to be written down, and the receipts kept in chronological order.

At intervals a partner or the accountant can go over the book, to ensure that all is correct. This will allow you to claim everything claimable against your tax, and you have the proof. Poor quality bookkeeping could cost you a significant amount of tax and if the Inland Revenue prove that you have kept incorrect records very expensive.

24 Expenditure

THIS is the part of making money which has little attraction, but is as important as any other. The old aphorism of 'a penny saved is a penny made' is true. What you spend at work, you cannot spend at home. It is very important to keep close control of outgoing money. Having said that, like all businesses, you need to continually invest. If you do not, you will slowly decrease your income and hence your spending power at home.

Expenditure can be divided into two types, that which creates a profit and that which does not. Typical of profit makers are practice nurses, minor surgery equipment, vaccines and smear equipment. The non-profit makers are there to service the profit makers. A receptionist will not often make you a profit directly, but if you do not have them, life is hard. If you are contemplating making a purchase for the practice, you need to ensure that it is needed, and that it cannot be done more cheaply in the long-term. For instance should you have fabric towels, paper towels or hot-air driers in the toilets? In the long term, hot-air driers may be the best buy despite the fact that they are the most expensive at the outset.

Maintenance

Remember that most long-lasting items need maintenance, particularly measuring equipment. There is not much use in having an audiogram or a spirometer if they are not accurate. Spend some money on keeping them calibrated. Buildings need maintenance. Make sure that you have a schedule for painting and other building care. It might be worth employing someone permanently either part-time or full-time to look after your buildings.

Suppliers

Most things are supplied by several suppliers. Compare prices or get your practice manager to do so for you. Beware of getting into long term contracts, as low prices now may become comparatively high in 5 years time. If you deal with one supplier for many things, haggle. Do not be shy of asking for discounts. They can be surprisingly easy to get. Stationery suppliers seem to be keen on special offers. If the offer is good, and it is for something which will not go out of date – perhaps envelopes – buy in bulk.

There should be a clear protocol covering who makes the routine purchases. It may be a partner or perhaps the practice manager. Drugs might be bought by your nurse, and stationery by the secretary. It is a road to expensive chaos having anyone buying what they want. You may want to have large purchases agreed at a practice meeting. However you decide to arrange your buying, make sure that whoever does it knows what they have to do, and the limits within which they can operate.

Having bought something, make sure that when it is delivered that it is what you wanted and also that the correct quantities are delivered. If you get a delivery of, for example, envelopes or tetanus vaccines they need to be checked by someone. If a receptionist is responsible for taking delivery, she should check off each article before signing the delivery sheet. Once the delivery sheet is signed, if there is any shortfall in quantities, it will probably be too late to argue. Keep the delivery sheet, and match it with the invoice. This job should probably be done by the practice manager. If they do match and the delivery is correct, the delivery sheet can then be disposed of.

Your next job is to pay the supplier. When you pay is up to you. Most firms, however, want their money within 30 days. If you intend to maintain your good name and a willingness of others to deal with you, reasonably prompt payment is required. You get most of your money at the end of each month, and it would seem reasonable to pay your bills then. This has several advantages. Firstly, it means that the bank is not having to carry your outgoings for any length of time, keeping your bank interest charges down. Secondly, as all cheques go out together, you can keep a tight check on what is being paid. One staff member can supervise the payments. So careless mistakes, like paying the same bill twice, are less likely to happen. Thirdly, if most of your outgoing and incoming money happens at the same time, you can arrange for your bank statement to be dated after it has all happened. This will allow you to keep a close check on your current financial position without having to have a big list of uncleared cheques.

Having paid your bills, keep the invoices in chronological order, with the number of the cheque used to pay written on the invoice. This helps your accountant to follow what has happened. It also eases your problems if there is a question about the invoice.

It is worth finding a corner where you can store all your old pay documents and invoices. We were in a situation recently where our ownership of an audiometer was questioned. With old invoices, we proved our argument.

Who signs the cheques? This is usually easy. It may be one or two partners. It might be worth having your practice manager as a signatory. You can put a limit on the size of cheques signable by a practice manager. Whoever signs will have the cheques scrutinized by the accountant.

Profit sharing

How you split the profits at the end of the month varies from practice to practice. It may not however be straightforward. One way or another you need to calculate your profit. That is your income minus your expenditure. Starting with the balance at the bank, subtract uncleared cheques and bills to be paid. Add practice income. Subtract an amount that you have agreed to leave to pay the Inland Revenue. You may also decide to subtract an amount to leave at the bank to cover outgoings such as petty cash which will be required before the end of the next month. You now have a profit – I hope! This can be calculated on a bit of paper, in a book, or if you are so inclined, on a computer spreadsheet or accounts package.

You may decide to split the profit as it stands. Remember that each partner does not necessarily get a cheque in proportion to his share of profit. He may have his own tax liability, his own superannuation liability and possibly contribution to his capital in the practice. These can be calculated easily by the accountant. A typical example is given below:

The practice of Drs Quinn, McGhee and Aitken

Drs Quinn and McGhee are on 37%, Dr Aitken, a newcomer, is on 26%. Dr Quinn has a tax liability for the year of £6,612, superannuation of £5,541 a low-cost endowment premium for the surgery of £3,659. His endowment premium is high, because he is paying it off over a short time. Dr McGhee has tax of £5,119, superannuation of £3,612 and endowment of £1,833. Dr Aitken's tax will be £2,437, superannuation of £1,862 and an endowment premium of £1,066. His tax liability is low, because he was unemployed for a part of the year for which the practice will be paying tax this year.

		Quinn	McGhee	Aitken
Capital account	30.4.91	2,636	3,186	2,295
Capital at	30.4.92	2,500	2,500	2,500
		136	686	(205)
Tax for the year		6,612	5,119	2,437
Superannuation		5,541	3,612	1,862
Low cost endowment		3,659	1,833	1,066
		15,812	10,564	5,365
Less capital equalization		136	686	(205)
Total liability		15,676	9,878	5,570
Monthly liability		1,306	823	464

The size of the cheque for each partner is now calculated

X is the sum to be divided

add to X the sum of the monthly liabilities (1,306 + 823 + 464) = 2,593

Dr Quinn gets
  X plus £2,593 × 37 ÷ 100 − £1,306 ((X + 2593) × 37/100) − 1306
Dr McGhee gets ((X + 2593) × 37 ÷ 100) − 823
Dr Aitken gets ((X + 2593) × 26 ÷ 100) − 464

So, if there was £5,000 to divide, Dr Quinn gets £1,503.41. Dr McGhee gets £1,986.41 and Dr Aitken gets £1,510.18. This may not seem fair to Dr Quinn, but he has higher outgoings than Dr Aitken.

The advantages of this way of splitting the profit is that each gets that to which he is entitled. The capital accounts stay within sight of each other, and no one ends the year by having to repay to the practice large amounts of money.

An alternative stratagem is to pay each partner a similarly calculated sum − but the same amount at the end of each month.

This has the advantage that everyone knows how much they will have to spend each month. The disadvantages are that if the total practice liability is not correctly estimated, the partners can significantly underdraw, or overdraw and have to pay the bank interest. One partner's liability may be inaccurately estimated, and he will have a big change in his income next year. Finally the other partners are in effect giving an overpaid partner an interest free loan.

There is a half-way house, where the practice splits the monthly profit, but has a safety net. In this case there is a minimum amount that is split at the end of any month, with the balance being met the next month. Each practice has different finances and will meet the problem in a variety of ways.

25 Joining a Practice

THE idea for this chapter came from a partner who felt that there was little advice for someone looking for a practice with the intention of joining as a partner.

Curriculum vitae

The first thing to do is to produce a good curriculum vitae. This needs to be typed and clearly set out. It has two purposes. Firstly it is to get you an interview and secondly to save time at interview. Make it look good. Start it with a heading and perhaps a photograph. A decent photograph may be all that is needed to lift you out of the bunch. Page 2 could have your date of birth, marital status, children, driving licence, etc. Below this comes your basic education to graduation, including any interesting times you have had at university. Where did you go on your elective? Page 3 will show your jobs since graduation, including a brief description and points relevant to general practice. You could end up with a little about you as a person, your hobbies and interests.

Applications

When replying to advertisements, select practices where you are prepared to work. This may be in one locality, groups, single-handed, cathedral cities or whatever. Do not apply to a practice in Islington if you want to live out in the country. If you are in doubt, ring up and ask. Most decent practices will at least be polite, and a telephone call may make you memorable when it comes to selection for interview.

Apply in accordance with the advertisement. If they ask for a handwritten letter of application, or photograph, enclose them. It has been known, when asked for a photograph, for someone whose interest was photography not to send one – a failure. You can ask, if you want, that if you are not selected, they send your expensive curriculum vitae back to you.

Interviews

Your brilliant application has got you an interview. If you cannot get there on the day, let them know immediately, and preferably by telephone – a letter may lose you the interview. Assuming that you can go, arrive in good time. Try to have a look around the area first.

At interview, sit relaxed. Do not slouch or sit at attention, and try to smile a bit. There may well be a preliminary interview, with a selection being asked back for a final interview. Answer the questions as best as you can. Remember that you are interviewing the practice as well. So ask them whatever you think is relevant. Whilst assuring them of your total commitment to the practice, you need to know what that commitment is. What hours will you be doing surgery, and also visits? When are you on call? If there any restriction on where you can live? What holidays will you get?

Remember that the partners in the practice are going to be your workmates for the next few years. Choose carefully, because it is much harder to get an interview and a job if you have broken up with a previous practice. Things can improve however if you do not achieve perfection first time. A newcomer gets the partners he is given when he starts, but he chooses those that come after. It is much easier to select people one at a time than getting a package.

You need to know your rewards. There will be a path to parity, this needs to be made clear. You also need to know approximately how much you will be earning. There may be practice capital which needs to be purchased. Many practices will allow a new partner to build up his partnership share. Practice premises may exist and if so you may be required to buy in. DO NOT PANIC. There are money lenders – banks and insurance companies – who are more than keen to help you out, and it is unlikely to be terribly expensive (*see* Premises). The practice may indeed have the solution set up for you already.

Assistantships

You may be asked to be an assistant for a while – usually 3 to 6 months. This is to allow them to look at you in action, and for you to look at them. This is not unreasonable, particularly as an assistant is likely to be a bigger drain on practice resources than a partner, because an assistant does not bring in a BPA. It is also expensive to dissolve a partnership. Indeed a partnership is probably in law a tighter relationship than marriage. Make the terms of an assistantship clear. The hours you work, the holidays you get and the amount that you will be paid. You will need to ensure that if things do not work out, you get to know early, so that you can start looking elsewhere. If that is the case you must be allowed time off for interviews.

Travelling expenses

If you have travelled a long way, travelling expenses may be available from the practice. Be careful how you ask, you do not want to appear as money-grabbing. Most practices will accept that long-distance travel for interview can be a major financial burden for a young doctor. Do not ask for reimbursement of a 50p bus ride.

Practice accounts

At interview, you can ask that if offered the job, you could look at the practice accounts and a practice agreement if it exists. Look carefully at them. Make sure that they are properly prepared. If the accounts do not cover a year, find out why. The answer may be simple, perhaps there was an earlier change of partnership. Look at the income, is this reasonable for the size of practice? Do they get a lot from non-NHS sources? – this may mean that they are stretched and having to do long hours of extra sessions. Are their expenses reasonable? Do they have a lot owing to the bank? If so, why? Again, there is likely to be a good explanation. Do all the partners have similar capital accounts? You can get a good idea of how a practice is administered by reading their accounts with care. It is unlikely that you will be allowed to look at the accounts unless the job is to be, or has been offered to you. You may or may not be allowed to show them to someone else, such as an accountant.

Remember that if you have left a job where you were an employee to go into general practice, you will now be self-employed. This will allow you a tax-free year, *see* The Practice Accountant.

Acceptance

If you are offered the job, before finally committing yourself, go and have a chat with the practice accountant. He will be able to clear any doubt that you have about the accounts and confirm your estimated income. He may be able to give you an estimated cash flow, month by month, for the next year. You can of course talk to your own accountant. This has the advantage that he is not currently working for a practice that you have not yet joined.

If you get the job, ask for a simple contract, setting out the basics. This would include when you start, the path to parity, the pay in any assistantship, the sort of hours that you will work any commitment to buy into the practice. The advantage of this if bilateral. The practice knows that you are going to turn up on the day you are due to start. You have a guarantee of employment that you can show to a bank manager or building society if you are needing a loan or buying a house.

A full practice agreement will usually follow you joining a practice. This takes time to prepare. It will need your ideas, and any special needs that you have. It will probably need to be drawn up by a solicitor, and will certainly need your solicitor to check it. The practice may need a certificate from an independent solicitor to confirm that the agreement conforms to basic requirements before the FHSA will recognize that a partnership exists.

Finally, enjoy your new job, you are likely to be doing it for the next 35 years.

Index

accountant 69–72
accounts, practice 72–9
anaesthetic fee 13
ante-natal care fees 11
anthrax immunization 32
architects 54
assistant, allowance for
    employment of 2
assistantships 96–7
associate allowance 2

basic practice allowance (BPA) 1–3

cervical cytology, target
    payments 28–9
cheques, signing 91
child health surveillance 21–2
community charge 49–50
complete maternity services fee 13
computer costs 65
confinement fee 12
contraceptive services 9–10
    to temporary residents 5
cost rent scheme 52–7
curriculum vitae 95

deprivation allowance 2–3
designated area allowance 1
diphtheria immunization 31
dispensing 37–9
drugs, purchase and storage 38

elderly patients, screening 20
emergency treatment 7
    to temporary residents 5–6
employment of staff 61–3
equipment, maintenance of 89
examination expenses for trainees 46
expenditure 89–93

financial year-end, date of 71

government departments, private
    work for 85

half-time 1
health centres 50–1
health promotion clinics 23

immediately necessary treatment 6
immunization 31
    children 25–8
    non-travellers 31–2
    travellers abroad 32
improvement grants 59
income tax 71–2
inducement payments 36
interviews 96–8
intrauterine device, fitting fee 9
invoices 91

job applications 95
joining a practice 95–8

leave payments 3
locum, allowances for 36, 67

maintenance of equipment 89
maternity leave for trainees 46
maternity medical services 11–13
    claims for payment 14–15
    completion of claim forms 15–18
    shared with another doctor 13–14
maternity payments 68
measles immunization 32
medicals, private 82–3
minor surgery 33
miscarriage fee 12
MMR 32

net profit percentage 78–9
netting-out 78
newly registered patients 20
night visit fees 7

Obstetric List 11
occupational medicine 83–5
out of hours services 7
outgoings 79
oxygen therapy services 39

petty cash 87
poliomyelitis immunization 31
postgraduate education
    allowance 41–2
post-natal care fee 12–13

practice accountant   69–72
practice accounts   72–9
practice protocol   20
practice staff scheme   61–3
premises   49
  community charge   49–50
  cost rent scheme   52–7
  improvement grants   59
  practice-owned   51–2
  in a private house   51
  privately rented   50–1
  refuse collection   50
  rent   50–2
  water rates   49–50
pre-school boosters   27–8
private patients   81–2
profit sharing   91–3

rates   49–50
refuse collection   50
removal expenses for trainees   45–6
rent reimbursement   50–2
retainer scheme   46–7
Review Body, and practice
  accounts   78
road-traffic accidents, emergency
  treatment at   6
rubella immunization   32
rural practice payments   35–6

screening   19–20
seniority payments   1–2
sharps, disposal of   50

sickness payments   67
staff, employment of   61–3
students, undergraduate   44
superannuation   78
suppliers   89–91
surgery, minor   33

target payments
  cervical cytology   28–9
  immunizations   25–8
temporary residents   5
  emergency treatment   5–6
  immediately necessary treatment   6
  and rural practice payments   36
termination of pregnancy fee   12
tetanus immunization   31
three-quarters time   1
trainees   45–6
trainers   42, 43–4
training   43–7
travellers, immunization   32
travelling expenses
  for interviewees   97
  in rural practices   36

undergraduate medical students   44

vaccination
  children   25–8
  non-travellers   31–2
  travellers abroad   32

water rates   49–50